ACEROLA

("Barbados Cherry" *Malpighia punicifolia*)

NATURE'S SECRET
TO FIGHT FREE RADICALS

LESLIE TAYLOR, ND

Bestselling Author of *The Healing Power of Rainforest Herbs*

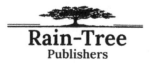

Rain-Tree
Publishers

The information and advice contained in this book are based upon the research and the professional experiences of the author, and are not intended as a substitute for consulting with a healthcare professional. The publisher and author are not responsible for any adverse effects or consequences resulting from the use of any of the suggestions discussed in this book. All matters pertaining to your physical health, including your diet and supplement routine, should be supervised by a healthcare professional who can provide medical care that is tailored to meet your individual needs.

Published by
Rain-Tree Publishers
Bullard, Texas 75757
www.rain-tree.com

ISBN: 978-1-7346847-2-8

Cover and Interior Production by Gary A. Rosenberg
www.thebookcouple.com

About the Rainforest Medicinal Plant Guide Series

This book is part of Leslie Taylor's Rainforest Medicinal Plant Guide series featuring the important medicinal plants of the rainforest that she has studied and used for more than 20 years. These guides provide factual, scientific, and vital information on how to use these powerful medicinal plants effectively to improve your health.

The author sells no herbal supplements or products other than books. The books in this series do not promote any specific brands or herbal supplement products. These definitive plant guides concern the plants and their researched effective actions and uses. The information in these guides is more extensive, complete, and unbiased than natural product companies who sell these plants as supplements can provide.

More information on Leslie Taylor's background, knowledge, and experience can be found on the Rain-Tree website (www.rain-tree.com/author.htm) See the Rain-Tree Publishers book page (www.rain-tree.com/books.htm) to learn when new plant guides in the series are released.

Contents

Introduction

What if there were just one supplement you could take that would make you look and feel younger, help you lose some weight, give you more energy, make you smarter, and decrease your risk of developing a host of chronic diseases? Recent research published on acerola shows that this amazing tropical fruit might just do that! This book will explain how and why.

When I wrote my rainforest book in 2005, *The Healing Power of Rainforest Herbs*, there were virtually no research studies published on acerola. All the health benefits for acerola were related to the high amount of vitamin C it provides. And it does contain an astounding amount of vitamin C—up to 10 times more than oranges when acerola is harvested when it's ripe and up to 50 times more when unripe fruit is harvested and used in natural and vitamin supplement products.

Research in the field of food science and nutrition has been focusing on the development of food products with higher nutritional values and the evaluation of foods for their health-promoting potential. As a result, the natural health industry coined the term "functional food" to describe foods that promote health and contain high levels of nutrients. In addition to fulfilling basic nutritional needs, functional foods provide additional physiological benefits, such as preventing or delaying the occurrence of chronic diseases. With acerola fruit being one of the richest natural sources of vitamin C ever known, acerola fruit and its products are in demand worldwide for the production of health supplements and in the development of functional food products. Acerola has well earned its "superfruit" designation in the natural health industry, and this book will tell you why.

You see, new research reveals that acerola is much more than the vitamin C it provides. What you'll learn from this book is the amazing "power of polyphenols" and the many health benefits these plant compounds can provide by fighting free radicals and relieving the oxidative stress and chronic inflammation they produce. Acerola delivers an incredible amount of these natural compounds, which have been proven repeatedly through research around the world to fight free radicals, relieve oxidative stress, reduce chronic inflammation, protect cells from damage, and even help repair cells that were damaged by free radicals. Polyphenols are now shown to be working in concert with the vitamin C in acerola to deliver important benefits that are far greater than vitamin C can provide alone, and they are key in avoiding many chronic diseases.

Tens of thousands of studies have been published in

the last five years confirming that free radicals and the chronic inflammation and cellular damage they create are now a cause or contributing factor to many diseases and conditions. Oxidative stress and chronic inflammation from free radical damage are playing major roles in the development or progression of a range of conditions, including type 2 diabetes and other metabolic diseases, clogged arteries and heart diseases, cancer, Alzheimer's disease, neurogenerative diseases, autoimmune diseases, and even obesity. The link is even more clear in age-related chronic diseases and in aging itself.

The recent growth in the knowledge of free radicals, and particularly types of free radicals called reactive oxygen species (ROS), is producing a medical revolution that promises a new age of health and disease management. This book will explain in easy-to-understand terms what free radicals are, how your built-in antioxidant system is supposed to keep these free radicals at healthy levels, the lifestyle and dietary factors that cause your built-in antioxidant system to falter, and how natural and effective polyphenol and vitamin antioxidants, like those found in acerola, can be the solution to restore your antioxidant system to optimal levels to keep you protected from disease.

Most important, this book includes a comprehensive consumer guide that provides important information about the acerola products available in the marketplace, how to choose the best product, and what dosages are most beneficial. As you will learn, not all acerola products are the same. You may not be able to find this in-depth information elsewhere, especially from an unbiased and reliable source that isn't trying to sell you their product.

We are currently in a healthcare crisis. Healthcare costs and health insurance rates have steadily risen as doctors' offices are jammed with patients trying to treat diabetes, heart disease, obesity, and a whole host of chronic diseases. You might be surprised to learn that many of these conditions are preventable. The main goal of this book is to share this new information that the underlying and contributing causes of these health problems are, in fact, caused by our failing antioxidants systems and how to naturally heal the natural processes in our antioxidant system to promote health and optimal wellness. Simple and natural health solutions such as these shouldn't be kept a secret. They should be widely shared to lower our healthcare costs while benefiting our overall health.

CHAPTER 1

What Is Acerola?

Acerola is the common name assigned to two species of tropical trees in the Malpighiaceae plant family—*Malpighia glabra* and *Malpighia emarginata*. Some sources even classify these two trees as the same species. Further confusion is generated because many botanists believe that *Malpighia glabra* should be reclassified as *Malpighia punicifolia*. This results in research being published and acerola products being sold using any one of these three scientific names. All three scientifically named trees are used interchangeably at this point and just called "acerola trees" or "acerola fruit" in commerce.

Description

Acerola is a large, bushy shrub or small tree growing up to 20 feet in height with an equal breadth. Acerola is best known for the abundance of bright red fruit it produces, which look similar to the European cherry. For this reason, acerola is also known as the Antilles, Barbados, Puerto Rican, or West Indian cherry tree. When ripe, the fruits are juicy and soft with a pleasant, tart flavor.

5

Although acerola fruit is commonly called a cherry, its odor and flavor are more like that of tart apples rather than cherries.

This pretty evergreen tree flourishes in warm and tropical climates, and its native distribution extends from South Texas through Mexico, Central America, and the Caribbean to South America and as far as Peru and Brazil. It has been introduced in tropical and subtropical areas throughout the world, including Cuba, India, China, Australia, Hawaii, Jamaica, and the Philippines as a cultivated fruit tree.

An acerola tree produces on average 44 to 66 pounds (20 to 30 kilograms) of fruit annually. Fruit yield depends on growth factors like soil conditions, rainfall, and adequate pollination by bees. The fruit is one-half to one inch (1.25 to 2.5 centimeters) in diameter with a three-winged seed inside, and unlike regular cherries, acerola cherries have three lobes to accommodate the three wings of the seed. The fruit starts out green and hard and changes to orange-red and then to a final bright red on ripening. Acerola trees produce and ripen its fruit quite rapidly— ripening occurs only three to four weeks after flowering. Trees can produce flowers and fruit continuously for eight to nine months out of the year, so acerola trees need to be harvested repeatedly as the fruit ripens. Although the sweetness of the fruit varies according to the variety and stage of harvest, most of them are quite tart and acidic. The tartness of the fruit comes from the very high amount of vitamin C it contains.

History

Acerola is thought to have been first introduced in the United States in the late 1800s, as acerola seeds from Cuba appeared in the catalog of the Royal Palm Nursery in Florida for the 1887–1888 growing season. In 1917, economic botanist, Hugh McCollum Curran, brought seeds from Curacao to the United States Department of Agriculture for evaluation. During that time, since acerola was very suitable to the growing conditions in Puerto Rico, the Puerto Rican government planted acerola trees around the island to help control soil erosion and, later, even handed out acerola tree seedlings to families during World War II to grow in their Victory Gardens for the tasty fruit it provided.

An explosion of interest in acerola occurred in 1945 when the School of Medicine, University of Puerto Rico, in Rio Piedras, determined that acerola cherries were the highest source of vitamin C ever recorded in an edible fruit. Worldwide publicity ensued, featuring the fruit under the Puerto Rican name of acerola, which has stuck ever since. This interest resulted in the Puerto Rican government establishing groves of acerola trees on the island and providing several thousand trees to be planted in schoolyards to supplement the vitamin C in children's diets. By 1954, there were 30,000 trees in commercial groves in Puerto Rico, several plantations were made in Florida, and 2,000 acres in Hawaii were planted with acerola trees. Acerola fruit pulp or juice was even added to commercial baby foods in the 1950s and 1960s to increase nutritional levels of vitamin C.

Over the ensuing years, demand for acerola waned since it was only marketed for its high vitamin C content. The vitamin C from a natural source like acerola could not economically compete with the much cheaper ascorbic acid synthetic products that were developed, which supposedly provided the same benefits with equal rates of absorption. It has only been recently that scientists are looking beyond acerola's vitamin C content to discover this superfruit's many benefits, and acerola is gaining in popularity again. Another driving factor in the renewed interest in more natural sources of vitamin C is growing consumer awareness of the sources of synthetic ascorbic acid found in dietary supplements today. Synthetic ascorbic acid is usually produced from fermented corn syrup, which can be extracted from genetically modified corn. Additionally, almost 80 percent of synthetic ascorbic acid used in food supplements today is produced in China with quality-control issues in that country coming under greater scrutiny by American consumers.

While there has long been commercial cultivation of acerola in some regions of the Americas, it is only in the last three decades that Brazil began to exploit it commercially. Currently, Brazil is the world's largest producer, consumer, and exporter of acerola products. Brazil commercializes it in the forms of juice, marmalades, frozen concentrates, jam, and liquors. Other acerola plantations of commercial importance are in Florida and Hawaii.

Traditional Uses in Herbal Medicine

Acerola juice is as common and popular in Brazil as apple juice is in North America. As a natural remedy in Brazil, a handful of fresh fruit is eaten for fever, colds, flu, and dysentery. Acerola fruit juice is also used in Brazil as an anti-inflammatory, an astringent, a stimulant for the liver and renal systems, and a diuretic to support heart function. It is also used to heal wounds. In Brazilian herbal medicine today, acerola is employed as a nutritive aid for anemia, diabetes, herpes, high cholesterol levels, liver problems, rheumatism, and tuberculosis, and during convalescence.

ETHNIC MEDICINAL USES OF ACEROLA	
Brazil	As a nutritive, astringent, anti-inflammatory, stimulant, and diuretic for anemia; for cardiovascular support, colds, diabetes, diarrhea, dysentery, fever, flu, herpes, high cholesterol, liver conditions, renal problems, rheumatism, tuberculosis, and wound healing
Guatemala	For anemia, diarrhea, colds, and flu
Mexico	For colds, fever, and flu
Puerto Rico	For anemia, colds, flu, and liver conditions
Venezuela	For breast conditions, colds, dysentery, hepatitis, and tenesmus

Acerola fruit is widely consumed as a food or beverage in the tropics where it grows. The ripe fruit, which is pleasant to taste despite being tart, is used in making jams, jellies and preserves, juice beverages, sauces, ice cream, pies, and wine and liqueurs. Acerola is so popular in Brazil, craft beer brewers are now adding acerola juice as a flavoring ingredient in their specialty brews.

Natural Compounds and Nutritional Value

Acerola is considered one the richest known source of natural vitamin C on the planet. Oranges provide 500 to 4,000 parts per million (ppm) of vitamin C, or ascorbic acid, whereas acerola has been found in tests to provide ascorbic acid in a range of 16,000 to 172,000 ppm. Acerola can contain up to 4.5 percent vitamin C, compared to 0.05 percent in a peeled orange. The vitamin C content of acerola varies depending on ripeness, season, climate, and locality. As the fruit begins to ripen, it loses a great deal of its vitamin content (and 50 percent of its vitamin C); for this reason, most commercially produced acerola targeted for dietary supplements is harvested while immature (green) or partially ripe (orange). For example, when fully ripe, the vitamin C content of the fruit ranges from 1,000 to 2,000 milligrams in 100 grams of fresh acerola and partially ripe fruit can have values as high as 4,500 milligrams in 100 grams. When acerola is freeze-dried (removing its 90 percent water content), the powders that are produced for the manufacture of supplements can deliver a whopping 15,000 to 20,000 milligrams of natural vitamin C in 100 grams.

Besides maturity, post-harvest handling and storage conditions can substantially impact vitamin C and the shelf life of acerola fruit. The information available in the field of acerola processing suggests that the vitamin C content begins to decrease about four hours after the harvest. Keeping the fruit shaded and cool during harvesting and then delivering it quickly into processing is the key to a nutrient-rich acerola product.

Although synthetic and food-derived vitamin C is substantially identical, fruit and vegetables are rich in numerous nutrients that may influence the bioavailability and uptake of the vitamin into the body. Two studies (one human and one animal) were published recently indicating this was true for acerola when they reported that the vitamin C in an acerola fruit powder was better absorbed and available to be used by cells (by 1.6 times) than the synthetic manufactured ascorbic acid vitamin C.

In addition to vitamin C, acerola also provides twice as much magnesium, pantothenic acid, and potassium as oranges. It also contains a significant amount of vitamin A (4,300 to 12,500 IU/100 g, compared to approximately 11,000 IU for raw carrots), as well as thiamine, riboflavin, and niacin in concentrations comparable to those in other fruits.

In addition to vitamins and minerals, acerola is also a rich source of other antioxidant chemicals, including cyanidins, anthocyanidins, terpenes, polyphenols, flavonoids, and carotenoids. Many of these chemicals are well known and studied, and a few have been discovered

FOOD VALUE OF ACEROLA FRUIT PER 100 GRAMS FRESH WEIGHT	
Water	91.41 g
Calories	32
Protein	400 mg
Fat (fatty acids)	300 mg
Fiber	1.1 g
Calcium	12 mg
Iron	0.20 mg
Magnesium	18 mg
Phosphorus	11 mg
Potassium	146 mg
Vitamin A	38 µg
Thiamine	0.020 mg
Riboflavin	0.060 mg
Niacin	0.400 mg
Vitamin C	1678 mg

that are unique to acerola. Most of these natural antioxidant chemicals have documented biological activity, and many of acerola's health benefits can be related to these powerful antioxidant compounds. Acerola also contains considerable dietary fibers (a kind of polysaccharide) with approximately 10 percent of the dry fruit being polysaccharide fiber, which include various plant pectins. Recently, pectic polysaccharides from acerola have been reported to have high antioxidant and anti-fatigue activities and comprise some of acerola's researched biologically active benefits. Pectin has also been shown in other research to help manage and lower cholesterol levels.

The fatty acids in the lipid (fat) fraction of the fruit include oleic, linoleic, palmitic, stearic, and linolenic acids. Carotenoids are yellow, orange, and red pigments present in many fruits and vegetables. Approximately 20 carotenoids are present in quantifiable amounts in the human body, and they play roles in health—mostly by synthesizing vitamin A. Of the six major dietary carotenoids found in humans, five are present in good supply in acerola fruits (beta-carotene, alpha-carotene, beta-cryptoxanthin, lutein, and zeaxanthin).

It has been well documented in acerola, as well as many other foods and medicinal plants that contain multiple natural antioxidant compounds, that there is a synergistic effect of multiple compounds working together, which provides much higher benefits than just a single compound like vitamin C working alone. The sum total is greater than any one part. The research discussed in the following chapters reveals that acerola has stronger antioxidant actions than vitamin C alone for this reason.

It is also well documented that multiple compounds working together eliminate the need to use high dosages of any one particular antioxidant compound. This can reduce side effects of single chemicals in high dosages. For example, vitamins A and E are effective antioxidants, but in very high dosages, toxicity can result. With acerola, the antioxidant action of the whole fruit is much greater than the action of either A or E in high doses but it is delivering its antioxidant action through the synergist action of many compounds working together. Many antioxidants present in lower amounts but working together raise the antioxidant capacity and negate the need to use too much of a single chemical, which effectively eliminates the negative side effects of taking high-dose vitamins or other single chemicals.

Thus far, more than 150 constituents have been identified in acerola. In addition to the vitamins and minerals mentioned, acerola contains many other active compounds, including aceronidin, antheraxanthin, apigenin, auroxanthin, benzoic acid derivatives, beta-carotene, beta-cryptoxanthin, beta-cryptoxanthin-5,6-epoxide, beta-cryptoxanthin-5,8-epoxide, cis-beta-carotene, cis-lutein, citric acid, dehydroascorbic acid, caffeic acid, caffeoyl hexoside, catechin, coumaroyl hexoside, coumaric acid, p-coumaric acid, cyanidin 3-O-rhamnoside, cyanidin, dehydroascorbic acid, dihydrocaffeoylquinic acid, diketogulonic acid, ellagic acid, epigallocatechin gallate, epicatechin, ferulic acid, furfural, gallic acid, hexadecanoic acid, isoquercitrin, isovitexin, kaempferol, kaempferol-3-O-beta-glucoside, kaemferol-3-rhamnoside, l-malic acid, limonene, lophirones, lutein, luteolin, luteoxanthin, malic acid, malonylapiin, malvidin chloride, neochrome, neoxanthin, pelargonidin, pelargonidin 3-O-rhamnoside, pectin, proanthocyanidin, protocatechuic acid, quercetin,

quercetin-3-α-O-rhamnoside, resveratrol hexoside, rutin, salicylic acid, syringic acid, sinapic acid, tartaric acid, violaxanthin, and vitexin.

I've used the word *antioxidant* several times in this chapter to describe various compounds in acerola. Before we go much farther, I want to make sure you really know what an antioxidant is and how it is capable of fighting free radicals and even what a free radical really is. The next chapter will tell you more about antioxidants, free radicals, and how vitamin C and other compounds found in acerola can help you maintain the delicate balance you need for healthy antioxidant levels and why that is so important.

CHAPTER 2

Free Radicals
and Antioxidants

The average American typically has some kind of basic knowledge (usually from advertisements) that "antioxidants fight free radicals," but most are unaware of exactly what a free radical is, why they need fighting, and how antioxidants work to "quench" or fight them. This chapter will explain the main types of free radicals, how they cause cellular damage, cellular dysfunction, and resulting illness, and the different ways specialized natural plant compounds with antioxidant actions (as well as vitamin C) can effectively reduce the number of free radicals in your body to promote health and avoid disease. Some of the powerful natural antioxidants discussed in this chapter can also stop cells from being damaged by free radicals and even help repair the damage they've already caused.

What Is a Free Radical?

There are two main types of free radicals: reactive oxygen species (ROS) and reactive nitrogen species (RNS). These substances are reactive because they are missing an electron. Our bodies are an oxygen-based system, as is most all life on the planet. Oxygen is an element indispensable for life. However, inside the body, some oxygen, with the help of a catalyst, splits into single atoms with unpaired electrons. Electrons like to be in pairs, so these atoms, called free radicals, scavenge the body for other electrons so they can become a pair. As they travel through the body in search of a new electron, they cause damage to cells, proteins, and DNA, and interrupt or change cellular signaling through a process called oxidation.

Consider what happens when you put a piece of untreated and unprotected metal outside in the elements or simply expose it to oxygen. Over time, the metal begins to rust. This rusting process is actually the oxidation of the metal—the chemical reaction of the metal to oxygen. ROS inside the body creates the same sort of rust-like reaction and damage as it comes into contact with unprotected cells. As another example: when the fats or oils we use to cook with are exposed to too much oxygen, over time they become rancid. The rancidity is actually oxidation of the fat molecules. When fat molecules (called lipids) in our bodies are exposed to too much ROS, they also rust or become rancid in a similar manner. For this reason, the oxygen-based free radicals (ROS) are much more damaging to our bodies, are the subject of much more research, are linked to many more diseases and conditions, and are what we will focus on in this book.

Free radicals, and specifically ROS, are a way of life. ROS are formed as a natural byproduct of the normal metabolism of oxygen, and they even play important roles in how cells communicate (called cellular signaling). Basically, free radicals are a byproduct of many different chemical processes going on simultaneously inside our wonderfully complex biochemical-driven bodies.

In addition to metabolizing oxygen, another large source of free radicals produced inside our bodies is the natural chemical process of how we metabolize our foods. Turning food into the cellular energy that all our cells need to function and even to survive is a complex biochemical process. Free radicals are waste products generated from various chemical reactions that occur in this natural food metabolism process. Therefore, how much we eat and what we eat can be significant factors that raise our ROS levels.

ROS are created inside our bodies through these natural processes, and catalyst substances in our environment can create even more ROS. External catalysts that generate free radicals can be found in the food we eat, the medicines we take, the air we breathe, and the water we drink. These substances include fried foods, high-fructose sugars, alcohol, tobacco smoke, pesticides, exposure to X-rays, chemicals and environmental toxins, and air and water pollutants. All these substances can significantly raise the levels of ROS and free radicals in our bodies to unhealthy levels, which results in oxidative stress. The levels of internally produced free radical also increase from immune cell activation, inflammation, mental stress, excessive exercise, ischemia, infection, cancer, aging, diabetes, and obesity, which takes us over the edge of balance and into the state of oxidative stress. ROS can also provoke inappropriate or overexpressed immune responses and cause autoimmune conditions, activate cancer genes, mutate healthy cells into cancerous ones, and greatly increase cellular-aging processes.

What Is an Antioxidant?

In the simplest of terms, the most basic definition of an antioxidant is a substance or molecule that lends one of its own electrons to a free radical that is seeking one to make a pair. When the free radical has a new set of paired electrons, it becomes a stable molecule and is no longer reactive and causing cell damage. Remember, free radicals are radical because they are missing an electron. This process of an antioxidant lending an electron is usually called "quenching free radicals."

Our Built-In Antioxidant System

Because ROS generation is a natural process, our bodies have a natural built-in antioxidant system that is supposed to disable these free radicals as they are created and keep them at healthy levels. This is a perfect example of one of the amazing ways our bodies maintain their delicate balance. Through other biochemical processes, our bodies produce chemicals that are the main antioxidants that make up our built-in antioxidant system. These include chemical enzymes called superoxide dismutase (SOD), catalase, glutathione peroxidase, and glutathione reductase, which are considered our first line of defense.

We also produce other substances that are non-enzyme antioxidants that participate in our built-in antioxidant system. These include chemicals we produce inside our bodies (and some of which are also sold as dietary supplements) such as lipoic acid, glutathione, L-arginine, coenzyme Q10, melatonin, uric acid, bilirubin, metal-chelating proteins, transferrin, and others.

Vitamin and Mineral Antioxidants

While these natural built-in antioxidants are main players in our antioxidant system, they need help from various vitamins and minerals that aid in the biochemical process to produce them, activate them, and help them do their job. These include vitamins A, E, and C, which we're supposed to be getting from the foods we eat. These three vitamins are the subject of thousands of studies on their antioxidant actions and the roles they play in the body and within our antioxidant system. Of these three vitamin antioxidants, vitamin C has been shown to be the most important to the system. And, as with many antioxidants, the combination of vitamin C with either A or E has shown to have higher antioxidant actions in much of the vitamin research. Vitamin C is also uniquely able to lend not one, but two of its electrons to free radicals. In addition, as discussed in the next chapter, vitamin C plays an essential role for our natural enzyme antioxidants to be produced inside the body and for them to do their job efficiently.

Also necessary to support our antioxidant system and its enzymes are the minerals selenium, manganese, copper, and zinc. These minerals play roles in the production and/or actions of our natural enzymes that fight free radicals. In fact, some of these minerals are capable of binding together with our enzymes, which increases their antioxidant actions and effects.

Plant Antioxidants

Plants, like humans, need oxygen to survive, and they also create their own species of reactive oxygen molecules (ROS) during their metabolism of the oxygen they breathe. For this reason, plants produce natural antioxidants in their cellular processes to keep ROS in check and at healthy levels, just as we do. These antioxidant plant chemicals are also an important component in a plant's built-in defense mechanisms (much like our immune system) that protect the plants from damage and stress of too much or too little rainfall/moisture, too much or too little sunlight, toxic metals and chemicals in their soil, high heat, intense sunlight, high humidity, and other negative growing factors. These natural plant antioxidant compounds also help heal the damage from browsing animals and insects chewing on them (the equivalent of wounds in humans) and help plants recover from various bacteria, mold, fungi, and plant viruses that damage them. In fact, many plant antioxidants are dually antioxidant and antimicrobial—capable of killing these bacteria and fungi species that try to harm them. Because plants are rooted to the ground and cannot flee from danger like we can, they create wonderfully complex biochemical defense mechanisms to fight those dangers and factors that might harm or kill them.

In addition to lending electrons, plant antioxidants can suppress the formation of ROS by inhibiting certain enzymes involved in their production. Plant antioxidants can also trigger the body's natural production of antioxidants and send them to cells that are being damaged by oxidative stress. Much as chemical messengers signal the immune system to send healing agents to the site of an injury, plant antioxidants signal the body's antioxidant system to send healing antioxidants to the site of oxidative stress, as well as encourage the production of more body-produced antioxidant chemicals.

Lastly, there are various metals in our bodies—including the iron circulating in our blood—that can oxidize and damage cells, much as ROS does. Some strong plant antioxidants, like those found in acerola, are capable of interacting with these metals and converting the body's metal pro-oxidants into stable products, much as they stabilize or neutralize free radicals, reducing oxidative stress.

Polyphenol Antioxidants

The main and most effective antioxidants found in plants fall into a category of well-researched plant compounds called polyphenols. Scientists have long known that the polyphenols in plants can benefit humans in many of same ways they benefit, protect, and heal plants. Polyphenols, which include the subcategories of phenolic acids and flavonoids, are the subject of a huge amount of research. More than 10,000 studies on plant polyphenols have been published in just the last five years. Not only do they have very strong antioxidant actions, but because they were uniquely created to help plants heal and repair damage, their actions in humans result in these antioxidants working in different ways than vitamin antioxidants and our own natural enzyme antioxidants, which are mainly quenching free radicals through electron sharing. The healing power of these polyphenols to positively affect our health is incredible, and thankfully more health-conscious consumers are learning of their many benefits.

Remember when coffee was once supposed to be bad for you and doctors told you to avoid it, mainly because of the heart-stimulant actions of caffeine? Then, suddenly, it was good for you. The same thing happened with chocolate and wine, which once were supposed to be avoided and are now considered almost health foods. What happened? It was all the new research on the powerful health benefits of polyphenols. Coffee, chocolate (especially dark chocolate), and wine (mostly red wine) are all significant sources of these powerful healing polyphenols. That polyphenols can overcome the negative effects of the caffeine in coffee, the high fat and calories in chocolate, and the alcohol content in wine, and still provide a net effect that is beneficial to our health speaks to the real power of these polyphenols.

In addition to coffee, wine, and chocolate, it is the fruits and vegetables in our diets that are our main source of healthy polyphenols. Polyphenols are also found in the oils of plant seeds and fruit seeds, and this is one of the reasons why olive oil is now widely consumed as a "healthy oil"—it is rich in polyphenols. The polyphenol content of the foods we eat vary widely based on many factors. And like vitamin C, some powerful polyphenols are water soluble and are very sensitive to heat. The high heat generated in cooking fruits and vegetables can significantly lower the polyphenol content, which is why many nutritionists recommend having lots of raw fruits and veggies in our diets—it's all about the powerful and beneficial polyphenols in these raw foods. Much more information on polyphenols are found in chapter 4.

Summary

In a perfect world, we'd be getting all the vitamins, minerals, plant antioxidants, and other vital nutrients we need from the foods we eat. We'd avoid foods that generate extra free radicals, and we'd maintain a healthy weight and a healthy antioxidant system as a result. More important, in doing so, we'd be providing all the necessary nutrients all these complicated biochemical processes need that are humming along silently behind the scenes—all of which keep us healthy and avoiding problems and diseases.

But let's face it. We don't live in a perfect world, and we are merely imperfect humans. That kind of scenario just doesn't describe the average American and or even the average human. I think that's why "food supplements" and "dietary supplements" were first created and related to that kind of terminology. Many of these products really *are* supplementing our diets with the necessary food nutrients that are missing from the foods we eat. Other dietary supplements are helping to overcome the problems from too many of the less-than-healthy foods and lifestyle choices we can't seem to give up.

This is why getting our daily needs of vitamin C is much better when it comes from a whole food source like acerola. Acerola contains a host of other beneficial natural plant compounds, including polyphenols, which naturally occur in the foods we're supposed to be eating in our daily diet. In addition to polyphenols, acerola contains fatty acids, carotenoids, and other plant compounds with effective antioxidant effects. These are the compounds that aid in the absorption and uptake of the vitamins and minerals in the fruit, provide synergistic actions to help vitamin C be a better antioxidant, and provide added antioxidant actions as well as host of other benefits and actions all on their own.

A single chemical, synthetically made ascorbic acid supplement just doesn't compare. While the vitamin C content may be equal between a synthetic vitamin C supplement and an acerola supplement, with acerola, you get so much more than just vitamin C. That being said, it is still always better to get the antioxidants we need from a diet rich in fruits and vegetables rather than from supplements. When we can't, a high quality acerola is a wonderful healthy alternative.

While vitamin C is one of the better known and researched natural antioxidants, it also provides many other functions for health, which will be discussed in the next chapter. You will learn why it is an essential vitamin required for many cellular functions for optimal health.

CHAPTER 3

The Health Benefits of Vitamin C

Vitamin C is essential for life, and yet, humans are among just a few types of mammals that cannot produce it within their bodies. Vitamin C must be obtained through our diet. Vitamin C, also known as ascorbic acid, isn't just an antioxidant. It is necessary for the growth, development, and repair of all body tissues. It's involved in many bodily functions, including formation of collagen, absorption of iron, production of immune system cells to fight infection, wound healing, and the maintenance of cartilage, bones, and teeth. In fact, this essential vitamin can be found residing in almost all the cells in our body in tiny amounts.

Vitamin C is an integral part of our built-in antioxidant system, including acting as a cofactor to support other natural antioxidant compounds our bodies produce that keep free radicals in check and at healthy levels. Vitamin C is the most abundant water-soluble vitamin antioxidant in our blood and tissues, and one of the most famous antioxidant supplements. It has been linked to many impressive health benefits, such as boosting over-all natural antioxidant levels, reducing blood pressure, reducing heart disease risk, protecting against gout attacks, improving iron absorption, boosting immunity, reducing dementia risk, and reducing cancer risk.

We have known about the importance of vitamin C for centuries. Deficient amounts of this essential vitamin cause a disease called scurvy. The word *scurvy* was first recorded in an English seaman's record in 1589. Sailors on long voyages with a lack of vitamin C–rich fresh fruits and vegetables in their diets were especially prone to developing this dreaded disease. It is estimated that more than 1 million sailors died during the seventeenth and eighteenth centuries due to scurvy.

The U.S. recommended dietary allowance (RDA) for vitamin C is 75 milligrams for women and 90 milli-grams for men. Just three acerola cherries would satisfy the RDA. However, this is generally regarded by most as the minimum amount necessary to avoid deficiencies. Much higher dosages of vitamin C are considered more therapeutic and beneficial by many natural health prac-titioners, and research has confirmed many benefits at higher-than-RDA dosages.

As vitamin C is water-soluble, it is not stored in the body, and therefore, there are few risks related to over-consumption. Whatever is not used by the body is simply excreted through urine. Humans also have a very small capacity for storing vitamin C; we can only hold about a thirty-day supply. Therefore, it is absolutely necessary to get our vitamin C from external dietary sources on a daily basis.

The Main Benefits and Actions of Vitamin C

The extensive research on vitamin C reveals the important health benefits discussed next. (See the reference section for a list of the research detailed.)

A Natural Antioxidant to Fight Free Radicals

Vitamin C is probably one of the best known and widely studied natural antioxidants. It has been the subject of human and animal studies over many years and well documented to reduce or neutralize free radicals and aids other natural antioxidants we produce to do their job more effectively. Vitamin C is typically used as a gold standard to compare the antioxidant abilities of other substances that are studied in several antioxidant laboratory tests.

Enhances Immune Function

One of the main reasons people take vitamin C supplements is to boost their immunity. The human immune system produces white blood cells called phagocytes. *Phagocytosis* is a medical term that describes the ingestion and destruction of bacteria, viruses, and other foreign invaders by these phagocytes. This is the chief defense mechanism of the human body against infection—our immune system's main role. The ability of phagocytes to carry out these activities has been shown to be associated with the presence of vitamin C in white blood cells. Vitamin C plays an important role in aiding these immune cells to function normally and kill microorganisms. Research indicates that raising levels of vitamin C in the body increases phagocytosis and helps the body fight infections more effectively. It has also been established through research to actually encourage the production of phagocytes and other white blood cells known as lymphocytes that also enhance immune function response. Moreover, vitamin C is helpful to strengthen the skin's immune defense system and helps wounds heal faster.

Promotes Collagen Production

Most people are aware that one of the main reasons our skin develops wrinkles as we age is a gradual loss of collagen in our skin. There is certainly no shortage of skin-care potions marketed to women to retard skin aging and decrease wrinkles by supposedly increasing skin collagen. Many of these anti-wrinkle potions even contain natural or synthetic vitamin C. However, you might be surprised to learn that collagen is about much more than just wrinkles. Collagen is actually the structural glue that holds us together as human beings. Collagen is the most abundant protein in mammals, making up from 25 to 35 percent of the whole-body protein content. It's the basic building block of all connective tissue that builds and strengthens not only skin, but teeth, bones, blood vessels, ligaments, and tendons as well.

Vitamin C is necessary to create collagen in our bodies in several different ways. Mostly, it is a cofactor (helper) for several important enzymes that actually make collagen. Without adequate vitamin C, these enzymes can't do their job and collagen production slows down. Most of the symptoms and ill effects of the vitamin C–deficient disease, scurvy, is due to a significant loss of collagen. Scurvy causes subcutaneous bleeding and bruising (due to weak blood vessels), poor wound healing (from poor skin collagen and immune function), joint pain and swelling (weak cartilage and ligaments), and thin hair and tooth loss (from a lack of collagen in those structures). The fatigue well noted in scurvy may well come from other enzymes that require vitamin C to produce L-carnitine. This is a molecule that converts fat into energy. Without enough of this enzyme, the body may not be able to burn fat, which will diminish fuel for energy production and cause fatigue as well as promote fat accumulation and weight gain.

Therefore, while promoting collagen production may well help keep our skin looking younger, it's hugely important to support the body's overall collagen production to keep bones, blood vessels, teeth, and the whole body strong. Making sure you have good vitamin C levels is necessary for this important aspect of wellness.

Promotes Healthy Aging

Researchers in Korea reported in 2015 that high dosages of vitamin C (1,250 milligrams daily) reduced the levels of advanced glycation end products (AGEs) in their human studies. AGEs are well documented to promote premature and regular cellular aging. They accumulate in the body (and skin) as we age and are a direct cause of many age-related chronic diseases and conditions. In addition, researchers examined links between nutrient intakes and skin aging in 4,025 women over age 40. They reported that higher vitamin C levels were associated with a lower likelihood of a wrinkled skin appearance, dryness of the skin, and a better skin-aging appearance. Taking vitamin C orally and using it topically has evidenced benefits to retard skin aging through the reduction of AGEs and oxidative stress, in addition to promoting collagen levels in the skin. In fact, it is the actual collagen in our skin that suffers the most damage from AGEs and free radicals, which causes the skin to age and wrinkle. See chapter 7 for more information on AGEs and the damage they cause, and how acerola may prevent AGE formation, disable them, and/or reduce their damaging effects.

Improves Mood Disorders

Vitamin C is believed to be involved in anxiety, stress, depression, fatigue, and our overall mood state. A significant amount of vitamin C is stored in the brain and helps regulate brain function. It has been demonstrated in human clinical trials in adults, adolescents, and children that oral vitamin C supplementation (1 to 3 grams daily) can elevate mood as well as reduce depression, stress, and anxiety. And, once again, having low levels of vitamin C due to poor diets has been reported to increase the risk of developing these types of mood disorders in all age groups.

Memory and Neurodegenerative Disorders

Vitamin C has been shown to participate in many different neurochemical reactions involving electron transport. Neurons are known to use vitamin C for many different chemical and enzymatic reactions, including the synthesis of neurotransmitters and hormones. Norepinephrine is an essential neurotransmitter that controls attention and memories in our brains. It's also responsible for delivering our biochemical response to physical and emotional stress, and it's made with the help of vitamin C.

Recent research has reported that higher doses of vitamin C are beneficial for various degenerative brain conditions such as Parkinson's disease, Alzheimer's disease, dementia, age-related memory loss, and others. Most of these benefits are attributed to the antioxidant actions of vitamin C and its ability to relieve oxidative stress, which is well known to be elevated in the brain in these types of neurodegenerative disorders.

Furthermore, high vitamin C intake from food or supplements has been shown to have a protective effect on thinking and memory with age. See more information in chapter 7 on acerola's ability to enhance memory, and chapter 5 on how free radicals can create oxidative stress in the brain to cause these disorders.

Helps Regulate Blood Pressure

The ability of vitamin C to help regulate blood pressure has been well documented. Researchers at Johns Hopkins School of Medicine analyzed 29 human studies and reported in 2012 that taking a vitamin C supplement (averaging 500 milligrams per day) can help lower blood pressure. It should be noted, however, that the drop in blood pressure levels in these studies were moderate and not strong enough to treat most hypertensive patients effectively as a stand-alone treatment. In people who had high blood pressure in these reviewed studies, systolic blood pressure (the top number in a reading) dropped by an average of nearly 5 points, while diastolic pressure (the bottom number) dropped by about 1.7 points. Once again, these benefits to modulate blood pressure are thought to be mainly attributed to the vitamin's antioxidant actions. The antioxidant activities of vitamin C may protect the lining of blood vessels from damage caused by oxidative stress and increase the availability of nitric oxide, a signaling molecule that helps relax arterial walls and reduce pressure.

Regulates Cholesterol and Prevents Clogged Arteries

Research reports that higher doses of vitamin C (1 to 3 grams daily) helps normalize and lower cholesterol levels. The antioxidant action of vitamin C also plays a role in preventing the oxidation of low-density lipoprotein (LDL) cholesterol. Oxidized LDL is one of the main components of arterial plaque. Having less oxidized LDL in our bloodstream helps prevent clogged arteries thereby naturally reducing the risk of heart diseases. As a result, many human studies report that consuming at least 500 milligrams of vitamin C daily may reduce the risk of heart disease. Additionally, research published in the *American Journal of Clinical Nutrition* found that those with the highest concentrations of vitamin C in their blood had a 42 percent lower stroke risk than those with the lowest concentrations.

Enhances Iron Absorption and Treats Anemia

Vitamin C supplementation has been used as a means of reducing iron deficiency and treating anemia as it aids in the absorption and uptake of iron from the diet. Vitamin C is able to convert plant-based sources of iron into a form that is easier for us to absorb. Research reports that taking just 100 milligrams of vitamin C may improve iron absorption by 67 percent. Researchers in China reported that a dose of just 50 milligrams daily effectively treated mild anemia in children as a stand-alone treatment.

Supports Male Fertility

Low vitamin C levels has been associated with male fertility problems. Vitamin C supplementation (at a minimum dosage of 500 milligrams daily) has been reported in several studies to enhance the production and mobility of sperm in both humans and animals. The fertility-enhancing action of vitamin C is mostly attributed to its antioxidant actions.

Benefits for Cold and Flu

Vitamin C has long been reported to be beneficial for colds and flu. Dosages from 2 to 4 grams and up to 8 grams daily have shown to ease symptoms of colds and flu and shorten the duration of infection. Lower dosages have shown little to no results in other research, which to some, makes the research seemingly inconsistent. However, if one compares the dosages used in all the research studies, it's clear this benefit is achieved with higher dosages. It's also possible that the immune system benefits discussed earlier that vitamin C increases phagocytosis plays a role in assisting the white blood cells to fight the infection more effectively. In fact, during the recent coronavirus outbreak in China, protocols were developed to treat hospitalized patients with high-dose vitamin C.

Benefits for Allergies and Asthma

Research reports people who took vitamin C regularly had fewer allergy problems, respiratory infections, and asthma attacks. A 1992 study found lower blood levels of histamine (which causes allergic reactions) in people who took 2 grams of vitamin C daily. In research conducted in Germany in 2018, high-dose vitamin C (intravenously) was reported to reduce allergy-related symptoms and act as an antihistamine.

Prevention of Glaucoma and Eye Diseases

Vitamin C has been shown to in several studies to lower intraocular pressure, which is elevated in glaucoma. Low levels of vitamin C has also been shown to increase the risk of developing glaucoma. Other research reports that vitamin C may provide benefits for age-related macular degeneration and cataracts. Most of the eye benefits reported for vitamin C are mainly attributed to the antioxidant actions of vitamin C and its ability to reduce oxidative stress and resulting damage in the eyes.

Adjunctive Support for Shingles

Shingles (a *Herpes zoster* infection) has been successfully treated with antioxidative substances like high-dose vitamin C for many years. Generally, vitamin C in high dosages, given orally or administered intravenously, has been shown in research to lessen the duration of the infection and reduce or prevent long-term nerve pain, which can persist after the infection. Antioxidants in general have been shown in research to protect nerves from oxidative stress and the damage it causes, which is a contributing factor in the nerve pain some people experience long after the virus causing the infection is gone.

Treats and Prevents Gout

Gout is an extremely painful condition caused by too much uric acid in body. Gout is actually a type of arthritis and occurs when excess uric acid crystalizes and deposits in the joints, causing pain and inflammation. Several human studies report that higher dosages of vitamin C (500 milligrams daily or more) can significantly lower uric acid levels and treat the condition, while other studies report lower dosages (100 to 300 milligrams daily) are beneficial in preventing future gout attacks. One study followed 46,994 healthy men over 20 years to see if vitamin C intake was linked to developing gout. Interestingly, their research revealed that people who took a vitamin C supplement had a 44 percent lower gout risk.

Cancer and Cancer Prevention

Over the past century, the notion that vitamin C can be used to treat cancer has generated much controversy. Vitamin C was first shown to be a potent, nontoxic, anticancer agent by Nobel Prize winner Linus Pauling in 1976. In his research, Pauling showed a 4.2 times longer survival time for terminal cancer patients who received 10 grams (10,000 milligrams) of intravenous vitamin C per day for 10 days, followed by 10 grams of oral vitamin C per day indefinitely. Subsequent research performed by others had some conflicts as well as different outcomes, and the use of vitamin C for cancer didn't fully catch on in mainstream medicine circles for many years.

However, new knowledge regarding how vitamin C works in the body and recent high-profile preclinical studies have revived interest in the utilization of high-dose vitamin C for cancer treatment. Studies have shown that intravenous vitamin C targets many of the mechanisms that cancer cells utilize for their survival and growth. The current mainstream thinking is that since the body's store of vitamin C is tightly controlled by several different built-in mechanisms, oral supplementation of the vitamin cannot achieve blood levels high enough that provide the ability to kill cancer cells. For this reason, most all human and animal research focusing on vitamin C and cancer today are using high dosages delivered intravenously. Intravenous vitamin C achieves blood concentration levels between 100 and 1,000 times higher than oral vitamin C can.

Cancer prevention, however, is a completely different story. Natural antioxidants (including vitamin C and other natural antioxidants found in acerola) have demonstrated in a huge body of research over the years to be beneficial in reducing the risk of developing cancer. Most of this research confirms that having a healthy built-in antioxidant system is the best method to prevent cancer.

One of the most compelling cases I am aware of for using vitamin C for cancer is from a friend and colleague, James Templeton. He is a long-term survivor of stage-5 melanoma who used high-dose intravenous vitamin C in the Pauling protocol many years ago when it was still rather controversial. His new book, *I Used to Have Cancer*, is a heartfelt account of his journey to healing and explains how vitamin C was integral to his cure and why he still takes high dosages of this important vitamin for prevention and wellness.

The Bottom Line

Vitamin C has gained a great deal of attention, especially lately—and for good reason. A recent study published in

Seminars in Preventive and Alternative Medicine looked at over 100 studies over 10 years which revealed a growing list of benefits of vitamin C. The lead researcher, Mark Moyad, MD, MPH, of the University of Michigan said in the publication: "Higher blood levels of vitamin C may be the ideal nutrition marker for overall health. The more we study vitamin C, the better our understanding of how diverse it is in protecting our health, from cardiovascular, cancer, stroke, eye health, [and] immunity to living longer." He also notes most of the benefits studied are achieved at higher dosages starting at 400 to 500 milligrams daily or higher.

Overall, vitamin C is linked to many impressive health benefits, and vitamin C supplements are a simple and cost-effective way to boost your vitamin C levels. With the rising number of Americans relying on processed, pre-prepared, and fast foods in their busy lives, lower nutritional levels, including low vitamin C levels, can be a result.

The recommended number of servings of fruits and vegetables is nine daily—a number most Americans struggle to meet. When you consider that vitamin C is heat sensitive and boiling or cooking can lower a food's nutritional value, including vitamin C levels, many people may be deficient in this essential vitamin without being aware of it. If you struggle to get enough natural vitamin C from the raw fruits and vegetables in your diet to maintain adequate nutrition, you should consider taking a vitamin C supplement.

Vitamin C Deficiencies

Smokers and low-income families are among those most at risk for vitamin C deficiencies. Regular alcohol consumption (and overconsumption) can also create vitamin C deficiencies. People (and especially children) with limited variety in their diets, people with malabsorption issues, and those with certain chronic diseases, long-lasting illnesses, and cancer may all experience vitamin C deficiencies. When illness strikes, the immune system responds naturally by increasing white blood cells to fight the illness. This can quickly deplete the body's store of vitamin C that these white blood cells require to do their job. If the illness is prolonged, vitamin C deficiency can result.

The first symptom of a vitamin C deficiency is unexplained fatigue. More subtle symptoms of vitamin C deficiencies (which can take months of chronic low levels to develop) include rough, bumpy skin, bruising easily, slow-healing wounds, painful or swollen joints, weak bones, bleeding gums, immune deficiencies, poor mood, thinning hair, and unexplained weight gain.

Acerola as a Solution

Whether you think you might have low levels of this important vitamin or you want to have optimal levels for the benefits detailed in this chapter, supplementing with acerola for your vitamin C needs is an option health-conscious people are turning to. A significant amount of natural vitamin C is delivered along with a host of other beneficial vitamin, minerals, and natural plant compounds that facilitate greater absorption and utilization by all the different cells and biochemical processes that require vitamin C to function properly.

Recent investigations suggest that ascorbic acid from natural sources is more readily absorbed by the human body than synthetically produced vitamin C. In a double-blind human study, it was found that vitamin C in acerola powder is 1.63 times more bioavailable in the human body than vitamin C synthetically produced. Other studies showed that infants consuming apple juice supplemented with acerola juice exhibited above average or average growth and development for their age and weight. Vitamin C levels in the blood were above average for all infants after the acerola juice was introduced in the diet. No allergic reaction was observed during this study, suggesting that acerola juice combined with apple juice is a good alternative to orange juice as a source of vitamin C in the diet.

There are many acerola products to choose from (see the consumer guide in chapter 8) that are reasonably priced, and many are now organic products. With more people trying to reduce GMOs in their diet, acerola is a great option to achieve optimal vitamin C levels for optimal health without the possible GMOs in synthetic chemical vitamin C supplements.

Remember, acerola is more than just the vitamin C it

contains. In the next chapter, we'll look at the other important natural antioxidant compounds found in acerola and how all these natural chemicals work together synergistically to fight free radicals, relieve oxidative stress and chronic inflammation, and interrupt the progression of chronic diseases.

CHAPTER 4

The Power of Polyphenols

In addition to a therapeutic level of vitamin C, acerola is a rich source of natural polyphenol chemicals that include anthocyanins, flavonoids, and phenolic acids. In fact, acerola delivers almost as many polyphenols as it does vitamin C, so it's an important aspect that adds to the benefits and actions of acerola far beyond its vitamin C levels. The amount of these polyphenols can vary in acerola fruit (and all fruits and plants), which will be discussed in this chapter. You'll learn why polyphenols are important and how they contribute to the documented actions and benefits of acerola for losing weight, better memory, higher energy levels, and looking and feeling younger.

You'll also learn that, of all known plant compounds, polyphenols have repeatedly been shown to be the most powerful for protecting against chronic diseases, including heart disease, clogged arteries, metabolic disorders like type-2 diabetes, dementia, Alzheimer's disease, Parkinson's diseases, and other degenerative brain diseases. Because they are the most protective, they are also the most preventative.

What Is a Polyphenol?

We've known about plant polyphenols for quite a few years, and they've been studied extensively. Over 80,000 research studies have been published on polyphenols since the mid-1980s, and research continues today at a fast pace. More than 8,000 different polyphenols have been identified thus far, and we continue to discover new ones, mostly in medicinal plants and novel tropical fruits.

Polyphenols are unique natural plant compounds that can be found in all plants and, typically, almost all parts of the plants—leaves, stems, barks, fruits, fruit peels or skin, seeds, and roots. Every plant contains a unique combination of polyphenols, which is why different plants and fruits, all rich in these substances, can have very different effects on the body.

All living things have inbred survival instincts. It is literally part of the cellular makeup of all species on earth. In highly mobile species like humans and other animals, the main survival instinct and mechanism is "flee, fight, or hide." Even bacteria and virus species have learned to flee or hide from immune cells and chemical agents attacking them, as well as to fight them by mutating or changing their own physical structure to defend against them. With stationary plants rooted to the ground and incapable of physically fleeing from danger, their survival instinct is controlled by wonderfully complex and rich chemical defense mechanisms that have evolved over eons. Plants have either created a chemical defense mechanism against what might harm them, or they have succumbed and become extinct. This is the mechanism the plants use to survive, grow, and flourish as well as to fight the many disease-causing organisms that attack them. Creating and utilizing polyphenols is one of the main mechanisms plants use to survive, grow, and flourish, to fight the many disease-causing organisms that attack them, as well as repair the damage they've caused.

Polyphenols are created in plants as a part of a plant's unique biochemical immune system and antioxidant system. These chemicals reduce free radicals and prevent or repair the damage caused by free radicals that the plants are exposed to. Oxidative damage in plants can be a result of less than perfect growing conditions, soil toxins and heavy metals, too much or too little water, too much or too little sunlight, and other negative conditions. Polyphenols are also the healing and repairing agents in plants' specialized "immune systems" to overcome and heal damage by insects and browsing animals, and to protect it from various microbes like plant viruses, bacteria, fungi, and mold.

This is why the type and number of polyphenols can vary widely in plants and the same plants can vary in polyphenol levels from one growing season to another. It really all depends on what types of damage and negative growing conditions the plants had to overcome by increasing its polyphenol content. The more stressful conditions, the higher the polyphenol content. It is also for this reason that wild-harvested plants usually have more polyphenols than cultivated plants. Growers of cultivated plants, like fruits and vegetables and even medicinal plants, control stress factors to their crops to increase harvesting yields . . . from proper irrigation, added soil nutrients, insect control, and even protection from intense sunlight. Controlling these factors will result in the plant needing to produce less stress-reducing and healing polyphenols.

These aspects also explain why tropical fruits like acerola usually have higher amounts and more diversity in their polyphenol content than cultivated fruits in the United States or Europe. The growing conditions in the tropics are just more intense and stressful. High humidity (which promotes more mold and fungi), intense heat and sunlight, and periods of monsoon-like rains followed by dry periods in the typical rainy-dry seasons of the tropics all contribute to the need of tropical plants to increase polyphenol production to protect themselves. And let's not forget about the bugs! Without a cold season to kill off crawling bugs as well as bacteria, viruses, and fungi, the diversity of pests that tropical plants are exposed to are *much* higher in the tropics than in temperate climates. When botanists say a particular plant has "adapted" to grow in the tropics, this adaptation is usually all about the plant's having increased its natural polyphenol production enough to survive in these more extreme growing conditions.

The consumption of exotic tropical fruits has gained in popularity in both domestic and international markets due to the growing recognition of their much higher nutritional and health-promoting effects. Fruit juices and dried fruit powders from acerola, acai, guava, graviola, camu camu, maqui berry, passionfruit, mango, and others are showing up in many functional foods and beverages as well as in dietary supplements in the natural products industry. And it's usually all about the powerful and high number of polyphenols these tropical fruits provide.

How Polyphenols Are Unique

The main feature that makes a polyphenol a polyphenol is its unique molecular structure, which usually makes them easy to identify. The manner in which the compound is put together molecularly facilitates a polyphenol to easily attach to and bond to other molecules and chemicals, oftentimes creating brand-new compounds. This unique molecular structure also makes polyphenols especially attracted to enzyme chemicals. However, rather than creating a new compound, they often bond to the enzyme and then disable the enzyme from performing its job, making them effective enzyme inhibitors.

For example, one of the reasons most polyphenols have antioxidant actions is that polyphenols are capable of binding with and interfering with two enzymes that are required in the complicated biochemical chain of events that creates a free radical, and especially ROS free radicals. Another good example is this: Some polyphenols are reported with weight loss or blood sugar–lowering actions because those polyphenols bond to and disable the digestive enzymes we produce during digestion that break down sugars and starches in our meals. If these enzymes don't do their job, then the sugar and starches (and their calories) are not broken down and absorbed (raising blood sugar levels and promoting weight gain), and they are eliminated undigested. Not all polyphenols can provide this benefit/action, but some can.

Polyphenols can bind with almost any type of compound—with sugars, with other plant chemicals, and even with each other. These types of new compounds are usually called derivatives or isomers of the chemical a polyphenol connected with. For example, there are two very common natural acids found in many fruits, vegetables, and medicinal plants called caffeic acid and quinic acid. When these two chemicals bind with one another, they create new chemicals that are basically combinations or bonds between these two plant chemicals. These bonds form isomers. One very well-known isomer of caffeic and quinic acids is chlorogenic acid (CGA). So far, more than 71 different CGA compounds have been reported and are widely distributed in plants. These various compounds are just slightly different derivatives of caffeic acid bonding with quinic acid, but actions, benefits, and absorption of these derivatives can be very different.

The binding action of polyphenols can happen inside plants to make more healing and antioxidant chemicals when the plant needs them, and these bonds can happen and new chemicals are formed inside our bodies during digestion. These types of chemicals are called metabolites—a product of metabolism. Unbelievably, while scientists have confirmed there are more than 8,000 unique polyphenols, they estimate that between 100,000 and 200,000 metabolites of polyphenols are created in plants, animals, humans, and even microbes like bacteria. This makes it harder for scientists to study since digestive processes are so unique, very difficult to create inside a test tube, are often different in laboratory animals than in humans, and are even different among individual humans. To make matters more complicated, some of these polyphenols are not easily digested, and they make it to the colon where we each have our own unique ratio of thousands of gut bacteria species that make up our gut microbiome. Landmark research over the last five years has shown that polyphenols interacting with bacteria in the gut microbiome make a whole host of new chemicals that contribute to many physiological functions. From chemicals that control our appetite, insulin sensitivity, fat storage, fat burning, and inflammation levels to the manufacture of neurotransmitters we need for mood, brain function, and much more, polyphenols are now thought to be the best way to modulate our gut bacteria to promote health.

We will probably never know the total effect polyphenols and their many isomers, derivatives, and metabolites have on promoting heath and treating diseases, but scientists agree, it's a fascinating subject that promotes rigorous ongoing research on these important natural compounds.

The Main Actions of Polyphenols

While every natural plant chemical can have unique actions and benefits, polyphenol compounds generally share some common properties and actions. These shared actions are detailed next.

Antioxidant Actions

Almost without exception, polyphenols are widely documented as strong antioxidants. Not only can they quench free radicals, but they have cellular-protective effects to protect cells and organs from the damaging oxidation and resulting cellular damage that free radicals cause. Utilizing their binding actions with enzymes, polyphenols interfere in the chemical chain of events that's required to make a free radical. Some polyphenols can also encourage the production of our own natural antioxidant enzymes to help address free radicals.

The powerful antioxidant nature of polyphenols has been demonstrated repeatedly in research to prevent or treat various diseases and conditions where oxidative stress is a factor in the development or progression of the disease—of which there are many. In addition, polyphenols are typically called "chain-breaking" antioxidants and are very important to add to vitamin antioxidants like vitamin C. When vitamin C lends an electron to a free radical, it becomes a pro-oxidant itself, and with two missing electrons, it can actually become a free radical, causing cellular damage until it is quenched by another antioxidant. When polyphenols lend electrons, they remain fairly stable and so prevent the initiation of further radical reactions. Polyphenols can also lend electrons to unstable vitamin C intermediates and "break the chain" reaction of vitamins turning from antioxidants to pro-oxidants to free radicals.

Anti-inflammatory Actions

The majority of polyphenols have shown some sort of anti-inflammatory action. Oftentimes inflammation is relieved or reduced simply by reducing free radicals and their damaging effects. You'll learn how oxidative stress causes chronic inflammation in the next chapter. Some polyphenols reduce inflammation by interfering in the biochemical chain of events our immune system uses to cause inflammation. This results in changes in the biochemical process where fewer pro-inflammatory chemicals are produced by the immune system and overall inflammation is reduced. This is considered an immune-regulating or immune-modulation action even though the end result is less inflammation. Again, more on inflammation in general follows in the next chapter.

Antimicrobial Actions

Many polyphenols have been shown to effectively kill bacteria, viruses, and fungi in humans, just as they do in plants. This can make some polyphenols and polyphenol-rich foods natural antimicrobial agents to aid in treating infections. These antimicrobial actions are also playing a role in the friendly bacteria (and not so friendly bacteria) in our gut microbiome. The antibacterial actions of polyphenols can kill off certain types of gut bacteria, yet paradoxically, other friendly bacteria are immune and use polyphenols as a food source (prebiotic) to increase in strength and numbers. Most of the gut microbiome research with polyphenols indicate they can modulate the bacterial species in a manner to treat obesity, help maintain a healthy weight more easily, reduce intestinal inflammation, and treat or prevent chronic bowel diseases such as irritable bowel syndrome and inflammatory bowel diseases.

Modulates Cholesterol

The majority of polyphenols play a beneficial role in the biochemical processes of how the human body processes fat in the diet. This benefit is largely attributed to the anti-oxidant action of polyphenols and preventing the changes in the biochemical process that occur from the actions of free radicals. The effects of free radicals can result in oxidized fat cells, causing deregulated cholesterol and triglyceride levels, the promotion of clogged arteries, and heart and vein damage, leading to high blood pressure and heart diseases. A classification of antioxidants called anthocyanins are the strongest among the polyphenols that benefit the heart and cholesterol levels.

Anti-Aging Actions

A significant number of polyphenols have shown the

ability to prolong the lifespan of laboratory animals in new anti-aging research. Again, free radicals are implicated in the overall aging process in both humans and animals. They can accumulate over the years in our bodies, resulting in state of chronic oxidative stress at old age. This affects not only our skin but also many internal cells, organs, and biochemical processes.

Inside most of our cells are organelles called mitochondria, and they play an integral role in biochemical processes going on inside our cells. Mitochondria, which are often called the powerhouses of cells, act like miniature factories, converting the food we eat into usable energy in the form of a chemical called adenosine triphosphate (ATP). ATP provides energy to fuel a myriad of cellular processes. If there is a biochemical process going on inside a cell, it is typically going on in the mitochondria.

Mitochondria are actually a significant generator of free radicals because free radicals are a byproduct of creating ATP. Each of our cells contain a little bit of vitamin C and antioxidant enzymes, and their role is to help deactivate these mitochondrial-produced free radicals. However, mitochondria can also be a target of free radical damage if our natural antioxidant system isn't doing its job effectively, leading to mitochondrial dysfunction. Research now reports that mitochondrial dysfunction is one of the root causes of aging, and it helps create a state of chronic oxidative stress in the elderly. As our cells age, mitochondria lose their ability to provide cellular energy efficiently and release more free radicals, including ROS, that harm cells.

Significant research on polyphenols has reported that these naturally strong and cellular-protective antioxidant compounds can treat and relieve mitochondrial dysfunction. Restoring mitochondrial function basically renews the cell and allows it to function like it did when it was much younger. This is one method by which polyphenols can deliver an anti-aging effect and why they can prolong life in animal studies. However, another significant factor in aging is the accumulation and damage of other free- radical–like substances called advanced glycation end products (AGEs). AGEs also accumulate in our bodies, cells, and organs as we age, and are considered to be the hallmark of cellular aging. The levels of AGEs in our bodies are now thought to directly relate to how well or poorly we age, as well as which age-related chronic diseases we are at risk for.

Again, the research on these powerful polyphenols are revealing that maybe the best natural compounds on the planet that are capable of reducing AGEs and protecting cells and biochemical processes from their damaging effects are polyphenols. Thousands of studies on polyphenols (including those found in acerola) report the anti-aging benefits these effective compounds can provide. See chapter 7 for more information on AGEs and problems they cause and why acerola was reported in research to provide these AGE-inhibiting and anti-aging benefits.

The Polyphenols in Acerola

As discussed in this chapter, polyphenol amounts in fruits and plants can vary depending on growing conditions. You'll also learn in chapter 8, the consumer guide, that polyphenol amounts can also vary based on harvesting and processing methods. Typically, polyphenol contents in acerola are shown to range from 100 to 150 milligrams in just one gram (1,000 milligrams) of freeze-dried acerola fruit powder. This is substantially higher than we can obtain from the regular fruits and vegetables in a normal diet, even those considered to be good sources of polyphenols.

For example, broccoli is considered a high-polyphenol vegetable that is being promoted as a healthy food to consume and is also sold as a functional food in various dried vegetable powder supplements. The polyphenol content of a dried broccoli vegetable powder has been shown to contain about 8 milligrams of polyphenols per gram of dried broccoli, which is far less than acerola's 100 milligrams. And to get the equivalent polyphenols by just adding fresh broccoli to your diet, several pounds daily would need to be consumed to equal just 1 gram of dried acerola powder. Also keep in mind that broccoli would need to be eaten raw, since the polyphenols in broccoli (and other nutrients like vitamin C) leach out or degrade when it's cooked in boiling water.

To date, acerola has been reported to contain more than 30 different powerful polyphenols. Since these natural compounds can bind to other chemicals during digestion, the total number of polyphenol compounds that result when we consume acerola can be much greater. The most significant (by volume) comes from a specific type of polyphenol called anthocyanins. In addition to providing antioxidant actions, anthocyanins play a role in fruits and vegetables as the main pigments that give them their red, blue, or purple colors.

The main anthocyanin polyphenols in acerola are cyanidin, pelargonidin, and malvidin, which regularly form the derivatives and isomers inside the fruit: cyanidin-3-rhamnoside, cyanidin-3-α-O-rhamnoside, pelargonidin-3-α-O-rhamnoside, pelargonidin-3-rhamnoside, and malvidin 3,5-diglucoside. Of the many phenolic acid type of polyphenols in acerola, p-coumaric and ferulic acids were identified as two major phenolic acids that acerola delivers in significant amounts. Much of acerola's researched actions are attributed to these anthocyanins and phenolic acids; however, it is well documented that all acerola's many polyphenols are working together synergistically, which results in the net effect of acerola's many benefits and actions.

The polyphenols acerola provides include aceronidin, apigenin, astragalin, benzoic acid derivatives, caffeic acid, caffeoyl hexoside, catechin, chlorogenic acid, coumaroyl hexoside, coumaric acid, p-coumaric acid, cyanidin, cyanidin-3-rhamnoside, cyanidin-3-α-O-rhamnoside, ellagic acid, epicatechin, epigallocatechin gallate, ferulic acid, gallic acid, kaempferol, luteolin, malvidin, malvidin

3,5-diglucoside, pelargonidin, pelargonidin 3-O-rhamnoside, proanthocyanidin, protocatechuic acid, rutin, quercetin, quercitrin, isoquercitrin, and resveratrol hexoside.

Different Polyphenols Means Different Actions

While all plants contain polyphenols, each plant has its own unique blend of these natural compounds that usually results in what each plant's overall benefits are. With more than 8,000 polyphenols to choose from in nature, the differences between the health benefits of different plants can be the specific polyphenols a plant contains. The next clue is to look at the actions of each polyphenol and their effective dosages to achieve a benefit. Some polyphenols work at extremely low dosages of just a microgram or two to derive a benefit, and others need much higher amounts. Even common spices like cinnamon and cloves, culinary herbs like oregano and thyme, and many medicinal plants are significant sources of beneficial polyphenols, which can be greater than those found in vegetables. And, as previously discussed, tropical fruits like acerola deliver a much greater amount of polyphenols than standard cultivated fruits.

Another interesting factor concerning polyphenols is their ability to target specific kinds of cells, enzymes, molecules, and organs. Some polyphenols have an affinity to target enzymes that result in weight loss, others target cells in the cardiovascular system, and still others target other types of cells, enzymes, or organs like the brain, endocrine system, liver, skin, etc. For example, the polyphenol profile of acerola is *much* different from the polyphenol profile of broccoli. Acerola contains anthocyanins (and a significant amount of them), while broccoli contains little to none of this specific type of polyphenol (unless you're eating purple broccoli). Anthocyanins have an affinity to benefit cells, organs, and enzymes in the cardiovascular system and will deliver those benefits much better than other polyphenols found in broccoli. For this reason, you'll see many more anthocyanin-rich purple, blue, and red fruits and vegetables being marketed as "heart-healthy" supplements than many other green vegetables or yellow fruits.

All polyphenols can fight free radicals almost equally, but the affinity to specific cell types usually affects where in the body these polyphenols migrate to and relieve and repair cellular oxidation and damage caused by free radicals. Oftentimes, the best way to determine these affinities is by testing the polyphenol-rich whole plant in animals and humans. *In vitro* testing just confirms the initial antioxidant ability of a plant to quench free radical inside a test tube. Scientists introduce the plant to known pro-oxidant free radical molecules in a test tube and measure how much of the plant substance was required to disable and neutralize the free radicals. While this confirms a plant's antioxidant ability, it has little to do with what actually happens inside the body (*in vivo*) and how these compounds get digested and where they go to interact with free radicals inside us.

For that reason, chapters 6 and 7 are all about the animal and human research that has been conducted on acerola. The research confirms where acerola's polyphenols are going and which cells and organs are achieving a reduction of free radicals and their damaging effects to provide health benefits. This kind of research is much more important and revealing than the many *in vitro* studies that have been conducted to confirm that acerola is an effective antioxidant.

The Takeaway

Hopefully what you've learned in this chapter is that polyphenols are important compounds that should be an essential component in your daily diet. This chapter has also revealed why vitamin C–rich *and* polyphenol-rich supplements like acerola are much more beneficial than a single-chemical, synthetic vitamin C supplement. I've always said that nature is a much better chemist than we, as mere mortals, could ever be. Most all plants that have significant levels of vitamin C also have significant levels of polyphenols, almost without exception. What we learned from the previous chapter is that while vitamin C is crucial to our built-in antioxidant system and very good at lending electrons to free radicals, you need other chain-breaking antioxidants like polyphenols to interrupt the normal process of vitamin C turning into first a pro-oxidant and then a free radical after losing its electron(s) to other free radicals.

So nature included high polyphenols in high-vitamin C plants, and so should we! If you're not getting enough vitamin C in your diet, you're probably not getting enough polyphenols either. Taking high dosages of synthetic vitamin C with a low-polyphenol diet may have the opposite effect and actually increase free radical production and oxidative stress instead of relieving it.

Before we review the actual research on acerola, the next chapter will explain how unrelieved high free radicals in our bodies promote diseases and conditions that could be completely avoided. This information will tell you why acerola provides a significant benefit in preventing diseases, as confirmed through research on this tropical fruit. It will also explain why poor diets and our typical "Western diet" is lacking in adequate polyphenols and can be full of free radical–producing foods. The changes in our average diet over the last 30 or so years has significantly increased the amount of preventable chronic diseases we are experiencing in our society as a whole. From obesity and cholesterol problems to heart and brain diseases and many more, in addition to the dwindling amount of fresh, raw, polyphenol-rich, and nutrient-rich fruits, vegetables, and whole grains in our diets, there's been a significant toll on our health.

CHAPTER 5

How Polyphenols and Antioxidants Prevent Disease

America is in the middle of a healthcare crisis. Not only are healthcare and insurance costs rising each year, the quickly rising number of people facing chronic diseases are packing doctors' offices at a rapid pace. That polyphenols and natural antioxidants like vitamin C can make a huge impact on preventing diseases almost sounds too simple and too good to be true. However, if you look at the radical changes that have taken place in our diet and lifestyles and relate that to the rise of chronic disease, it's not so hard to understand.

Over the last 50 years, the average American diet has changed significantly. If one takes a step back and looks at the overall broad changes, the most significant factor seen is that our diets consist of food that's lacking in essential vitamins, minerals, and antioxidant polyphenols and includes far too many types of food that promote free radical production and/or harm our built-in natural antioxidant system. The end result has our protective antioxidant system in a state a crisis, which has contributed to the significant rise in chronic diseases we're faced with today. This chapter will discuss how our diet has changed our antioxidant levels and explain how you can avoid the most common chronic and age-related diseases to promote a longer and heathier life with an antioxidant-rich diet or antioxidant-rich supplements like acerola.

The Western Diet

The average Western diet is low in polyphenols, and the so-called advancements we've made in how we process food over the years seems to be all about removing polyphenols from the food we eat. For example, the largest supply of polyphenols in grains are in the coating of the grain seeds. We went from eating lots of healthy polyphenol-rich whole grains to consuming processed white flour and white rice with the seed coating removed. That is how whole wheat is processed into white flour—they remove the darker-colored polyphenol-rich coating of the seed. This has lowered our polyphenol intake levels significantly.

Starches

The Western diet contains lots of starchy processed foods using white flour. Cakes, cookies, white bread, starchy sweet cereals . . . we are consuming way too many calories from starches in our diet that are lacking in any polyphenols. It isn't surprising that the main vegetable eaten in the Western diet is starchy potatoes. The popularity of french fries isn't going away anytime soon! Most of the polyphenols in potatoes are in the skin, which is usually removed during processing. The high starch in the Western diet increases overall calories of average meals, and when you combine that with less physical exercise in our more sedentary lifestyles, it ends up as one of the causes of weight gain and obesity. But as you'll learn soon, just having less polyphenols in your diet or having chronic oxidative stress is another important cause of weight gain and obesity in the rapidly expanding world population—expanding in weight faster than in population numbers.

Fats

Instead of natural butter and animal fat (lard) comprising most of the fat we used to consume, hydrogenated vegetable oils and margarines replaced them. Butter is a source of polyphenols and essential fat-soluble vitamin antioxidants, as well as important essential fatty acids that act as antioxidants and anti-inflammatory agents. Even animal fats contain polyphenols and beneficial fatty acids.

Additionally, infusing today's manufactured fats and oils with hydrogen to extend their shelf-life promotes more reactive oxygen species (ROS) free radicals to form as our bodies try to digest them. Frying foods repeatedly in the same hydrogenated vegetable oil (think fast-food french fries and fried chicken) actually creates free radicals in the oil, so eating these types of fried food raises our free radical levels because we are actually consuming more free radicals.

So instead of our dietary fats providing natural antioxidants to fight free radicals, the fats we are consuming today contain free radicals and/or promote the creation of free radicals. In fact, it is the polyphenol profile of olive oil that makes this oil a great "healthy oil"—olive oil is full of polyphenols. It's also why butter is making a comeback as being a "healthy fat" again and why you should consider adding butter and olive oil to your diet to replace some of the margarine and hydrogenated oils you currently consume. See the section "Cardiovascular Diseases" later in this chapter to learn how the antioxidant nature of these natural saturated fats can help prevent heart diseases rather than increase heart risks due to higher saturated-fat consumption.

Sugars

White sugar and high-fructose corn syrup (HFCS) have replaced the brown sugar, honey, molasses, and other natural sugars we used to consume. The one thing in common among the natural sugars we no longer eat regularly is their polyphenol content. Processing sugarcane or beets into white sugar removes all the polyphenols, which usually taste bitter. The actual sugarcane and beet plants are full of polyphenols; the processed white sugar from these plants has none.

More alarming, scientists now report that consuming HCFS can slow the production and action of our natural enzyme antioxidants, which we need to keep free radicals in check. You'd be amazed at how quickly your free radical levels would decrease if you just eliminated the sodas and fruit juices with HFCS from your diet. When I read this new research, I wondered whether high-HFCS foods should bear a warning label just like cigarettes do. Both generate an unhealthy level of free radicals with inevitable health issues. While consuming too much of any kind of sugar has established negative health effects, the high level of white sugar and HFCS is one of the main negative effects in the Western diet that increases our risks of developing chronic diseases.

Fruits and Vegetables

The Western diet is also very low in raw fruits and vegetables. As a society, we are consuming way too much processed and fast foods in our busy lives, and these types of meals are severely lacking in fruits and vegetables. Fresh fruits and vegetables are supposed to be the main source of polyphenols in our diet. Researchers looking at this aspect of diet and nutrition in the modern diet reported that the main source of polyphenols in the Western diet now comes from coffee and chocolate. Polyphenols from vegetables in the diet came in dead last. Even drinking wine (which contains polyphenols) was higher than vegetables in their analyses. This is mostly because we just aren't eating the daily recommendation of nine servings of fruits and vegetables a day—and usually far less than that. And if one or more of those servings in our diet is a fruit juice loaded with HFCS, it doesn't really count since it will do more harm than good for our antioxidant system!

While coffee and chocolate do contain a significant amount of polyphenols (the polyphenol profile is similar in both sources), those who consume them are still missing many other important beneficial polyphenols from other foods sources. And let's face it, fruits and vegetables are also an important and main source of the vitamins and minerals in our diets that we need to be healthy—chocolate and coffee are pretty lacking in that department. In fact, the researchers studying the natural antioxidants in modern diets noted that when you look at all antioxidants consumed in modern diets, those coming from vitamin-type antioxidants (vitamins A, C, and E) represented less than 10 percent of the total natural antioxidants consumed. We simply cannot rely on just coffee and chocolate (or wine) alone for the polyphenols we need—not if we want to stay healthy.

The Net Results of Poor Diets

Basically, the hallmark of a Western diet is the lack of essential nutrients we need, including natural vitamins and polyphenols that keep our antioxidant system humming along and doing its job of keeping free radicals in check. Havoc ensues when our antioxidant system falters or we're consuming too many empty calories from foods lacking in these nutrients and which promote more free radicals instead.

Before we discuss what damage and diseases oxidative stress causes, you need to know about chronic inflammation. You may be surprised to learn that one of the main deregulations and effects that free radicals cause is the level of inflammation in our bodies. Oxidative stress and chronic inflammation go hand in hand and have surfaced as the "root of all evil" when it comes to chronic diseases. Free radicals and inflammation are uniquely intertwined since inflammation promotes the creation of free radicals and free radicals promote inflammation—they are reacting together in a self-perpetuating cycle that leads to the development of multiple diseases.

The Inflammation Connection

Inflammation seems to be the new buzzword in the health industry, in both conventional and natural health circles—as well it should be. Tens of thousands of researchers and scientists around the world have documented the major role that inflammation plays in health and disease, and their discoveries are staggering. We now know that inflammation can be a cause of or a contributing factor to a wide range of disorders, including almost every chronic disease. There are even new anti-inflammatory diet and recipe books being published these days, teaching readers how they can modify their diets to reduce inflammation. And, if you read them, most promote excluding foods that promote the generation of free radicals (the wrong kinds of fats and sugars) and adding lots of polyphenol-rich fruits and vegetables.

Some books and researchers talk about the connection

between free radicals and chronic inflammation, and some only focus on the inflammation factor. However, what everyone should be learning is that the main cause of chronic inflammation is the negative effect of too many free radicals damaging cells in many parts of the body. Free radical damage causes inflammation. Taking anti-oxidants instead of anti-inflammatories can well treat the underlying causes of chronic inflammation in addition to the diseases they cause instead of just treating the inflammatory symptoms. Once you get your antioxidant system healthy and humming along as well as reduce your free radical load, you don't need to take anti-inflammatories to just treat symptoms. As a naturopath, I've long looked for root causes of diseases instead of relying on mainstream approaches of focusing and treating symptoms instead.

When most people think of inflammation, they think of the body's temporary response to injury and infection—a response that can be painful but is an essential part of the body's healing process. Unfortunately, not all inflammation is beneficial to the body. To understand why, we have to look at the difference between acute and chronic inflammation and how free radicals cause chronic inflammation.

Acute Inflammation

Acute inflammation is where our immune system shines. When we suffer an injury, such as a sprained ankle, chemical messengers known as cytokines are released by the damaged tissue and cells at the site of injury. These cytokines act as "emergency signals" that send out more of the body's immune cells, hormones, and nutrients. Blood vessels dilate and blood flow increases so that the healing agents can move quickly into the blood to flood the injured area. This inflammatory response is what causes the ankle to turn red and become swollen. As the healing agents go to work, the ankle is repaired, and the inflammation gradually subsides.

When you get a cut or wound, the same thing happens. Special white blood cells (known as natural killer cells) along with clotting and scabbing nutrients rush to the area to prevent infection, stop the bleeding, and form a scab. Again, the body's response causes redness and inflammation around the wound, but it is a sign that your immune system is at work protecting you from infection and healing the injury. Without this natural inflammatory response, wounds would fester and infections would abound.

Chronic Inflammation

Long-term, or chronic, inflammation is different from acute inflammation, and it's where our immune system and our natural inflammatory processes can cause problems. Chronic inflammation is also called persistent, low-grade inflammation because it can produce a steady, low level of inflammation throughout the body. This condition has been proven to contribute to many diseases, and research suggests it may cause some common chronic diseases such as diabetes, heart diseases, and even aging.

Low levels of inflammation can be triggered by a perceived internal threat—just as an injury triggers acute inflammation—even when there isn't a disease to fight or an injury to heal. This can activate the body's natural immune response, and inflammation is the result.

Free Radicals: The Leading Cause of Chronic Inflammation

The cellular damage caused by free radicals is the main perceived threat in our bodies that activates the immune system to cause inflammation. When healthy cells become damaged or begin dying from free radical damage, the body triggers the immune system to start the inflammatory process in an effort to repair or remove the cells. Because free radicals are distributed throughout the body, and the cellular damage is occurring cell by cell wherever a free radical interacts with a healthy cell, the inflammatory response spreads throughout the body. The cell-by-cell damage is smaller than damage caused by injury or infection, so the inflammation response is much smaller. This results in low levels of chronic inflammation throughout the body as the immune system tries to do its job of cleaning up or repairing free radical–damaged cells.

Unfortunately, when an imbalance occurs between the production of free radicals and the ability of the body to counteract these substances' negative effects, a negative feedback loop can be generated. In some cells and systems in the body, oxidative stress causes inflammation, and the inflammation can trigger the generation of even more free radicals. Then these additional free radicals create more oxidative stress, which causes more inflammation—a vicious cycle is created, and everything become chronic. It is important to understand that this process may have a detrimental effect on every one of our cells and in many of our complicated internal biochemical processes in different organs. This negative cycle can continue silently, usually without any outward symptoms or signs, causing us significant risks of developing chronic disease without even knowing.

While free radical damage can be the biggest cause of chronic inflammation, it's certainly not the only cause. But that's where polyphenol antioxidants can play a huge role and a greater one than vitamin antioxidants and our own natural enzyme antioxidants can. Most all polyphenols have antioxidant *and* anti-inflammatory actions. Polyphenols work in several ways to reduce and relieve inflammation, not just through reducing free radicals. Whether a problem is created by oxidative stress or chronic inflammation, polyphenols can be effective—if you pick the plants that have the right polyphenol combinations and profiles.

Diseases Caused by Oxidative Stress and Chronic Inflammation

Tens of thousands of research studies have been published on chronic inflammation and oxidative stress and the roles they play in numerous diseases. We now know that inflammation and oxidative stress can be a cause or a contributing factor to a wide range of diseases, including almost every chronic disease. From heart diseases, diabetes, Alzheimer's disease, and cancer to high cholesterol levels, autoimmune diseases, and even obesity—chronic inflammation and oxidative stress are playing significant roles. Many of these studies reveal that when you reduce oxidative stress and chronic inflammation, it has a beneficial impact on these conditions. Better yet, if you manage your levels of oxidative stress and chronic inflammation with polyphenol antioxidants, you can avoid developing these many conditions. Polyphenol compounds with antioxidant and anti-inflammatory actions have surfaced in all this research as the most important natural plant compounds available to us that have the ability to help prevent these diseases.

Obesity

New research indicates that obesity is actually a chronic inflammatory disease, and the fatty tissues of overweight individuals are inflamed and suffering from oxidative stress and immune cell damage. When fat cells and fatty tissues are damaged by inflammation and oxidative stress, they do not produce enough of certain natural metabolic chemicals that are required to reduce inflammation, store and burn fats, maintain insulin sensitivity, and support a healthy weight.

Scientists have now discovered more than 80 adipokines that are secreted by fat cells, many of which have known metabolic actions. Research has increased significantly on these natural fat-produced substances and their roles in obesity, diabetes, heart diseases, and other disorders since 2010. New knowledge about these substances and their roles have encouraged the development of new drugs targeting this metabolic system in the treatment of obesity, metabolic diseases, and heart conditions.

Since our fatty tissues and fat cells expand as we gain weight, all these fat-secreted deregulations and resulting inflammation and oxidative stress increases as our fat increases. You don't have to be obese either; just gaining some extra weight can start the process and head you down the road to deregulations. These deregulations make it much harder to lose weight, and some can make it virtually impossible to lose weight. Adipokines also help regulate functions in the heart and how we process sugar and insulin. Obesity-caused adipokine deregulations are now the main link of why obesity significantly increases our risks of developing type 2 diabetes and cardiovascular disease.

We once believed that many of us gained weight as we aged mostly because of reduced activity levels. New research is reporting that the accumulation of free radicals and advanced glycation end products (AGEs) as we age may be the cause of deregulations that promotes weight gain and makes it harder to maintain a healthy weight. Plants that contain strong antioxidant compounds, including acerola, have been reported in many studies to treat obesity and promote weight loss by reducing free radicals and lowering oxidative stress and chronic inflammation, which repair the deregulations that occur in our fat-produced metabolic adipokines.

A significant amount of research has been conducted in humans and animals on many different polyphenols that report weight-loss benefits and actions. The main mechanisms of actions reported is the reduction of oxidative stress, AGEs, and chronic inflammation, in addition to some polyphenols' ability to lower the calories in foods by blocking digestive enzymes that break down fats, sugars, and starches.

Cardiovascular Diseases

Adipokines produced in our fat cells control how we regulate our blood pressure and fluid balance, create new blood vessels, and how well our hearts contract to regulate blood flow. The direct deregulations of adipokines in fat cells created by obesity is now considered a main reason that, when we gain too much weight, we are at greater risk for developing heart problems.

In addition to fat deregulations, free radicals are particularly damaging to the cells in the heart and cardiovascular system because they are actually circulating in our bloodstream and are in constant contact. Thousands of studies report the mechanisms by which free radicals and the oxidative damage and inflammation they cause can contribute to the development of clogged arteries, high blood pressure, peripheral vascular disease, coronary artery disease, cardiomyopathy, heart failure, and cardiac arrhythmias.

Free radical damage is also the main reason people who smoke cigarettes have *much* higher risks for developing cardiovascular diseases. Cigarette smoke actually contains free radicals, and the chemical reactions smoke creates in the lungs generates significantly more free radicals. Chemicals used in e-cigarettes and vaping solutions are poorly studied for possible free radicals they might produce in the lungs. The recent reports of lung inflammation and lung cell death (the hallmark of free radical damage) doesn't bode well for the safety of these poorly studied chemicals going into your lungs. If you stop smoking, free radical production in your body will drop dramatically and you'll reduce the risk of free radical damage to your heart and cardiovascular system to prevent heart diseases.

Polyphenol antioxidants, including those found in acerola, are the subject of a substantial body of research documenting their actions and benefits to the cardiovascular system and their ability to prevent heart diseases. Many human, animal, and *in vitro* studies report that polyphenols exert beneficial effects on the vascular system via the increase of antioxidant defenses and reduction of oxidative stress. These beneficial effects include lowering blood pressure, improving endothelial function, inhibiting platelet aggregation (which reduces blot clots), reducing low-density lipoprotein (LDL) cholesterol oxidation, and relieving chronic inflammation by reducing inflammatory responses. The link between polyphenol consumption and the reduction of heart disease risk is well established and widely accepted.

Diabetes and Metabolic Diseases

Type 2 diabetes is also categorized as a chronic inflammatory disease that is associated with oxidative stress and insulin resistance. The increased production of reactive oxygen species (ROS) or a reduced capacity of the ROS-scavenging antioxidants can lead to abnormal changes in intracellular signaling and result in chronic inflammation and insulin resistance. Prevention of ROS-induced oxidative stress and inflammation can be an important therapeutic strategy to prevent the onset of type 2 diabetes and well as diabetic complications and co-occurring diseases.

New research also reveals that fat cell–produced adipokines play important roles in glucose metabolism and insulin resistance. It is established through human research that adipokines are deregulated in people with diabetes, and these deregulations are one of the underlying reasons obesity or just being overweight increases the risk of developing type 2 diabetes. Since many of these adipokine deregulations can be remediated with substances that reduce inflammation and oxidative stress, polyphenols have evolved as natural substances that can treat or prevent diabetes.

The initiation and progression of diabetes can also be linked to higher AGE levels in the body and the cellular damage, generation of additional free radicals, and inflammation these AGEs cause.

A significant body of research represents important advances related to influence of polyphenols and polyphenol-rich diets on preventing and managing type 2 diabetes. This research reveals that the main methods of actions polyphenols utilize to prevent diabetes include protection of pancreatic beta cells against glucose toxicity; anti-inflammatory and antioxidant effects; inhibition of digestive enzymes, which decrease starch conversion and sugar absorption; and inhibition of AGE production. Anthocyanin-type polyphenols have also been reported to exhibit antidiabetic properties by reducing blood glucose and HbA1c levels as well as improve insulin secretion and resistance in human and animal studies.

Neurodegenerative Diseases and Brain Disorders

Neurodegenerative disorders such as dementia, Parkinson's disease, and Alzheimer's disease represent an increasing problem in our aging societies, primarily as there is an increased prevalence of these diseases with age. These and other neurodegenerative disorders appear to be triggered by multifactorial events; however, oxidative stress and inflammation in the brain underlie most all neurodegenerative diseases and disorders. Neurons in the brain are frequent targets of oxidative stress, and the resulting cellular damage can lead to cell death and deregulation of chemical processes in the brain.

Studies looking at dietary factors and brain disorders report that regular dietary intake of polyphenol-rich foods and/or beverages has been associated with 50 percent reduction in the risk of dementia, a preservation of cognitive performance with aging, a delay in the onset of Alzheimer's disease, and a reduction in the risk of developing Parkinson's disease. Some polyphenols (including some anthocyanins found in acerola) have been reported to reduce the neurodegeneration associated with the accumulation AGEs during normal and abnormal brain aging.

Research also suggests that some polyphenols (particularly anthocyanins) are able to cross the blood-brain barrier; thus, these polyphenol compounds are likely to be candidates for direct neuroprotective and neuromodulatory actions. Polyphenols are considered to be neuroprotective because they provide a defense against many underlying causes of neurodegenerative diseases, namely oxidative stress, neuroinflammation, protein aggregation, metal toxicity, and mitochondrial dysfunction.

There is also a growing interest in the potential of polyphenols to improve memory, learning, and general cognitive ability. Human studies suggest that polyphenols may have a positive impact on memory and depression, and there is a large body of animal behavioral research to suggest that anthocyanin polyphenols are effective at reversing age-related deficits in spatial working memory, in improving object recognition memory, and in modulating inhibitory fear conditioning.

Liver Diseases

The most leading causes of liver diseases are oxidative stress, lipid peroxidation (the oxidation of fats by free radicals), chronic inflammation, and immune response deregulations. Natural polyphenols have attracted increasing attention as potential agents for the prevention and treatment of liver diseases. Their striking capacities in relieving oxidative stress, lipid metabolism, insulin resistance, and inflammation put polyphenols in the spotlight for the therapies of liver diseases as well as for the prevention of liver diseases. Numerous studies on polyphenols and polyphenol-rich medicinal plants report the liver-protecting ability of these substances. Thousands of animal studies report that cellular-protective polyphenols can protect the liver from just about anything scientists give the animals—liver-toxic drugs, toxic doses of aspirin and alcohol, and other substances or diseases like diabetes, which are known to cause liver damage.

Age-Related Eye Diseases

Oxidative stress and inflammation play a critical role in the initiation and progression of age-related eye abnormalities such as cataracts, glaucoma, diabetic retinopathy, macular degeneration, and even the autoimmune eye disease Sjögren's syndrome. Therefore, natural plant chemicals with proven antioxidant and anti-inflammatory activities, such as carotenoids and polyphenols, could be of benefit in preventing and treating these diseases. Several carotenoids and polyphenols in acerola have shown significant preventive and therapeutic benefits against these eye conditions in animal and human research.

Summary

When you understand the importance of polyphenols and how they can prevent many diseases, it's not all that difficult to understand why we're in such a health crisis with the significant rise in chronic diseases we're experiencing today. Our diets no longer contain the natural polyphenols that are necessary to support our antioxidant defenses to keep our oxidative stress and inflammation levels within the healthy levels, and illness ensues. More than 50 percent of the American population is overweight with rising levels of chronic inflammation and oxidative stress, 48 percent have some type of cardiovascular disease led by the increasing number of people with hypertension, and more than 100 million American adults are now living with diabetes or prediabetes. Metabolic syndrome, a prediabetes condition that usually leads to diabetes, now affects 30 percent of the U.S. population.

If your diet is much like the standard Western diet, you should be choosing the dietary supplements you need to overcome the deficiencies that are increasing your risks for ill health and disease. Choosing whole-food sources of polyphenol-rich foods to add to your diet is the best strategy, and, second to that, adding whole-food supplements like acerola that are rich in essential nutrients as well as in significant levels of beneficial polyphenols can help prevent deficiencies that lead to the preventable chronic diseases discussed in this chapter. For that reason alone, consumers should consider getting their daily vitamin C from acerola rather than from a single-chemical, synthetic vitamin C supplement.

Now that we've reviewed all the information on how the power of polyphenols contribute to the treatment and prevention of many diseases, it's much easier to understand how an exotic tropical fruit like acerola can live up to the claims that it can help you look and feel younger, lose weight, give you more energy, make you smarter, and decrease your risk of developing a host of chronic diseases. The next chapter will look at the actual research that has been conducted specifically on acerola in humans, animals, and test tubes that confirms these benefits and actions.

CHAPTER 6

The Benefits of Acerola
in Fighting Free Radicals

In previous chapters, you learned that keeping free radicals at low and healthy levels is very important to promote overall health and avoid disease. You also learned that the high amount of vitamin C and significant amount of antioxidant polyphenols delivered in acerola make it a perfect choice to keep your free radical levels in check and support your in-house antioxidant system so that it can do its important job. The only other necessity is to look at the actual research on acerola's strong antioxidant action. This chapter will briefly review 50-plus published research studies from researchers around the world confirming this superfruit's antioxidant actions, which far surpass that of most other fruits, vegetables, and medicinal plants.

The Research on Acerola's Antioxidant Actions

As mentioned, more than 50 studies have been published to date confirming acerola's antioxidant actions. There are several tests utilized to measure the antioxidant potential of plants and their compounds. In plant research, a test called the DPPH radical scavenging assay is the most extensively used to determine the antioxidant value for plant samples since it's inexpensive, quick, and accurate. This test has been the most accepted model for evaluating the free radical scavenging activity of any new drug. DPPH is a free radical that reacts with plants or compounds able to donate an electron and render it into a stable molecule.

Scientists place the plant or compound sample in a test tube with the DPPH and measure how much of the plant is required to stabilize the free radicals and how long it takes to do so. Interestingly, the standard reference compound most researchers use to compare the plant sample against is vitamin C since it is the best known and most widely researched natural antioxidant compound. Acerola's very high vitamin C content, combined with its high polyphenol content, results in this tropical fruit measuring, in DHHP tests, with the highest free radical–scavenging actions of all polyphenol-rich plants.

For example, another high-polyphenol tropical fruit that has gained in popularity in the U.S. natural product market that comes from the Brazilian Amazon is açai (*Euterpe oleracea*). Since about 2005, açai has been widely marketed for the polyphenol antioxidant actions it provides for weight loss, memory enhancement, disease prevention, and anti-aging benefits. It is a popular ingredient in many functional foods and beverages in the marketplace today for its antioxidant benefits. However, if you compare the DHHP test results for acerola with açai's test results, you'll see acerola wins the free radical–scavenging ability in this test . . . hands down. It took more than five times the amount of açai to stabilize the same amount of DHHP radicals as it took acerola, and acerola stabilized the free radicals in 10 minutes compared to 120 minutes for açai. Other researchers comparing DHHP-tested antioxidant actions reported that acerola exceeded the antioxidant actions of green tea, red wine, pomegranate, vitamin C, and vitamin A—all promoted to fight free radicals. For way too many years, consumers believed acerola was just about its high vitamin C content. Hopefully, growing consumer awareness of acerola's superior results to fight free radicals will increase the use and demand for this superfruit in the future.

Another test measuring antioxidant actions of natural substances that is growing in popularity is called an ORAC (oxygen radical absorbance capacity) assay. The ORAC assay is different in that the free radical used in the test (called AAPH) is a ROS-generating free radical that is commonly found in the human body. Additionally, AAPH is reactive with both water- and fat-soluble substances, so it can measure total antioxidant potential better than DHHP in plant samples with water- and fat-soluble antioxidant compounds. Usually the standard control used for comparison of antioxidant abilities for this test is fat-soluble vitamin E, rather than water-soluble vitamin C. Another test can be used called a FRAP assay, which measures the ability of a substance to address the oxidation of metals in the body, which is a significant ROS generator. And yet another antioxidant test that's used is called an ABTS assay (also known as Trolox equivalent antioxidant capacity, or TEAC).

When antioxidant actions are tested in animals or humans, other tests are performed that measure the actual hydroxyl and superoxide radical levels in the bloodstream, and/or nitric oxide (a free radical), and lipid peroxidation (oxidation of fat) levels. When these levels are reduced following the administration of a drug or natural substance, antioxidant actions are confirmed.

Acerola has been tested in every assay method known to measure antioxidant actions, and the bottom line is that this tropical fruit has strong antioxidant actions in all test methods. Most researchers in these many studies attribute acerola's strong antioxidant actions to the synergy of many polyphenols working in concert with vitamin C rather than any one single chemical or compound. Researchers also note that acerola has considerable amounts of carotenoids, some of which are converted to vitamin A when digested. Vitamin A is one of the main natural vitamin antioxidants our built-in antioxidant system needs to fight free radicals, and this is also playing a role in acerola's overall antioxidant abilities. Finally, acerola contains significant amounts of pectin (a type of polysaccharide) that has also demonstrated strong antioxidant actions (among other actions) and is contributing to this tropical fruit's overall strong antioxidant abilities.

Cellular-Protective Actions

Among the antioxidant actions documented by research are studies that report acerola's ability to protect cells and organs from oxidative stress. Researchers in Nigeria showed that acerola and several of its active antioxidant chemicals could protect liver cells from high dosages of liver-toxic acetaminophen in 2016. In that same year, researchers in Brazil reported that acerola protected cells from mutation and reduced side effects of a chemotherapeutic drug for cancer (known to harm and mutate healthy cells) in mice.

Metal ions such as iron can induce DNA damage and oxidative stress, and a different Brazilian research group reported that acerola fruit juice completely protected laboratory animals from DNA damage from high dosages of iron when they pretreated the animals with the juice in a 2016 study. Another group of Brazilian researchers reported that acerola protected thyroid cells of rats from damage and mutation from a radioisotope iodine drug that's normally used to test thyroid function and is known to cause cellular damage. In a 2018 study, acerola juice protected the brain cells of adult and aged rats from chemicals meant to replicate aging in the brain, in addition to repairing aged brain cells in older rats. This action might prove helpful for brain cancer patients undergoing radiation and chemotherapy to protect heathy brain cells from damaging free radicals caused by the therapy. In 2002, Japanese researchers reported that pretreating lung cells with acerola prevented the mutation of cells into cancerous ones when exposed to chemicals known to cause lung cancer.

In a test-tube study published in 2017, researchers in Ecuador reported that acerola protected skin cells from induced oxidative stress damage by decreasing cell death, reducing intracellular free radical levels and lipid (fat) and protein damage, and improving in-house antioxidant enzyme activities and mitochondrial functions.

In an *in vivo* study with mice, researchers also reported acerola's ability to repair or reverse oxidative stress damage and published their results in 2015. Mice were fed a high-sugar and high-fat "cafeteria" diet until they were obese. After inducing obesity in the mice, they fed the mice acerola for a month, and researchers noted that the acerola supplementation led to a partial reversal of the diet-induced DNA damage in the blood, kidney, liver, and bone marrow. The most recent research on acerola's cellular-protective actions was published in 2020 and focused on acerola's polysaccharides instead of poly-phenols. These researchers in China reported the poly-saccharides had antioxidant actions and protected the liver from fatty deposits and oxidative stress that leads to non-alcoholic fatty liver disease. They reported that acerola polysaccharides prevented fat from depositing in the liver, reduced inflammation and oxidative stress in the liver, and promoted enhanced mitochondrial function in liver cells.

The last significant thing to note in all the antioxidant

studies on acerola is the comparison of antioxidant abilities related to the ripeness of the fruit and the processing or manufacturing of the fruit into products suitable for foods and dietary supplements. The bottom line in these many studies is that polyphenols, vitamins, polysaccharides, and resulting antioxidant capabilities are much higher in unripe and partially ripe freeze-dried acerola fruits, followed by dehydrated partially ripe fruits, and lower still in processed fruit juices and pulps with ripe acerola. The values are the lowest in spray-dried fruit extracts, which uses heat and alcohol. More on this subject is found in the consumer guide in chapter 8 since it directly relates to how to find a good acerola product.

Summary

Acerola's strong antioxidant actions have been confirmed repeatedly, making this superfruit a wise choice for reducing chronic inflammation and oxidative stress as well as protecting you from chronic diseases and other conditions. When you support your built-in antioxidant system with acerola, you're supporting your overall health and wellness. You'll find a listing of the antioxidant and cellular-protective research conducted on acerola in the references section of this book if you are interested in reading about this further.

CHAPTER 7

More Benefits
and Uses of Acerola

With acerola's powerful antioxidant and anti-
inflammatory actions, it's not surprising that it
has been the subject of other research on diseases and
conditions where inflammation and oxidative stress play
major roles. Many of the benefits previously discussed for
vitamin C and/or polyphenols have been researched and
confirmed in acerola. This chapter reviews the science
and research conducted on acerola for diabetes, obesity,
healthy aging, brain function, and more. See the reference
section for a listing of all of the published research discussed in this chapter.

Anti-Aging and AGE-Inhibitor Actions

As discussed in previous chapters, aging has been associated with a chronic low-grade inflammatory state as well
as increased oxidative stress. It is widely accepted that
reactive oxygen species (ROS) in many cells accumulate
over our lifespan and lead to a state of chronic oxidative

stress at old age. Low-grade inflammation caused by oxidative stress is also now strongly linked to much higher risks of developing age-related memory loss, dementia, and even Alzheimer's disease. Acerola's strong antioxidant actions to fight free radicals, including ROS, and relieve oxidative stress and chronic inflammation are at the core of acerola's ability to promote healthy aging.

However, another huge area of anti-aging research over the last 10 years indicates that reducing advanced glycation end products (AGEs) in the body provides anti-aging benefits. AGEs are harmful compounds that are formed when protein or fat combines or bonds improperly with sugar in the bloodstream. This process is called glycation. These improperly bonded compounds can travel throughout the body and cause a host of problems, including chronic inflammation, cellular damage and cell death, and the interruption of cellular signaling. AGEs also encourage the creation of ROS, which generate oxidative stress and more inflammation. In fact, AGEs and ROS are uniquely intertwined. For an AGE to be created inside the body, the protein or the fat that creates the bond has to be oxidized first, usually by ROS. Therefore, having higher ROS levels means having more AGEs. Once an AGE is created, the damage and inflammation it causes results in the formation of more ROS, and a negative cycle is established.

AGEs and the damage they cause are now linked to cellular aging and premature aging inside the body and in various organs. Over a dozen different AGEs have been identified in the human body, and about half are known to accumulate with age in skin cells, affecting collagen production and promoting wrinkling and thinning of the skin. The rest of the AGEs can start accumulating in other organs and in the bloodstream, causing aging and cellular damage in the heart and cardiovascular system, kidneys, liver, and brain, resulting in chronic age-related diseases in these organs.

The link between AGEs and age-related diseases was recognized as early as 2001, when medical researchers at the University of South Carolina reported in the journal *Experimental Gerontology* that "they [AGEs] accumulate to high levels in tissues in age-related chronic diseases, such as atherosclerosis, diabetes, arthritis and neurodegenerative disease. Inhibition of AGE formation in these diseases may limit oxidative and inflammatory damage in tissues, retarding the progression of pathophysiology and improve the quality of life during aging." Recently, measuring AGE levels in individuals over age 60 has been proposed as a possible new blood test to monitor healthy aging and to enable the early detection of age-related diseases.

If we want to age well, or even slow aging, one of the best ways to accomplish that is to effectively manage our AGE levels. Some polyphenols have shown to be effective AGE-inhibitors in many different studies and acerola contains eight well-known polyphenol compounds with documented AGE-inhibitor actions. Three of these compounds are delivered in a significant amount in acerola fruit and have been the subject of research on the anti-aging actions of acerola. Researchers in Japan reported that three polyphenol compounds (cyanidin-3-α-O-rhamnoside, pelargonidin-3-α-O-rhamnoside, and quercetin-3-α-O-rhamnoside) they extracted from acerola and tested individually strongly inhibited the formation of AGEs. Their study reported that acerola and these three isolated compounds inhibited AGEs much better than the chemical compound normally used for this purpose in research (aminoguanidine).

Anti-Obesity and Weight-Loss Actions

As discussed earlier, obesity is associated with a decrease in antioxidant capacity, higher levels of damaging free radicals, and resulting chronic inflammation, and many studies have shown beneficial effects of antioxidant supplementation in treating obesity. Metabolism, the process through which the body converts food into the energy needed by every cell in the body to function, is controlled by a collection of glands known as the endocrine system. Metabolism involves a chain of events. As part of this chain, the hypothalamus, an area at the base of the brain, produces a chemical messenger called thyrotropin-releasing hormone (TRH). TRH is sent to the pituitary gland, where it regulates the production and secretion of thyroid-stimulating hormone (TSH). TSH is then sent to the thyroid, where it triggers the production of triiodothyronine (T3) and thyroxine (T4), two of the main chemicals responsible for metabolizing food into cellular energy.

One of the causes of the growing obesity problem we are seeing in America is an increase in thyroid dysfunction—specifically, hypothyroidism (or underactive thyroid), which slows metabolism. Actually, the underlying cause could be a dysfunction of any of the three organs—the hypothalamus, the pituitary gland, or the thyroid—involved in producing hormones that metabolize food into fuel. All these organs can suffer from oxidative stress, resulting in chronic inflammation and mitochondrial dysfunction, leading to improper function in one or more of these organs. This, in turn, can mean that rather than being turned into fuel, more food is being stored as fat. Brazilian researchers reported in 2013 that acerola protected the thyroid of rats from damage by a thyroid-damaging drug that increases ROS in the thyroid, so acerola's ability to reduce ROS in the thyroid was confirmed in animals. Other studies confirm that obesity can cause abnormalities in the hypothalamus as well, usually from DNA damage and mitochondrial dysfunction caused by ROS.

Another group of Brazilian researchers studied the anti-obesity actions of acerola in laboratory animals they fed a "cafeteria diet" to induce obesity and published four studies between 2014 and 2017. Personally, I would describe the diet they gave the animals in these studies as a "junk food diet" since it included chocolate crackers and cookies, soda, bacon or cheese chips, marshmallows, sausage hot dogs, and other snack foods like Doritos and a type of Italian bologna with lumps of fat in it (mortadella) along with their normal animal chow. The diet was certainly full of high-starch, fat, and sugary junk foods! And it's not surprising that such a diet turned healthy mice into unhealthy, obese mice quite quickly (in just 13 weeks).

These researchers confirmed that the obesity and bad diet led to oxidative stress that caused DNA damage and mitochondrial dysfunction in the hypothalamus, blood, kidney, liver, and bone marrow. After they gave acerola to the obese mice, they noted that it relieved the oxidative stress to the organs and partially reversed the DNA damage with acerola's strong protective and repairing antioxidant actions. The 2017 study reported that acerola fruit juice possesses anti-obesity actions by modulating chemicals and processes in the hypothalamus and brain in laboratory animals to increase overall metabolism and to release fats stored in cells. Two of these studies also noted that acerola was interfering with the metabolism and uptake of starches and sugars. Acerola interfered with the digestive enzyme (alpha-amylase) that breaks down starches into sugars, resulting in lowering the amount of calories absorbed in the junk food diet. This benefit was reported by other researchers studying the antidiabetic actions of acerola and by other researchers, which will be discussed later in this chapter.

The 2014 study reported that acerola relieved the oxidative stress and inflammation in the fat cells and fatty tissues of the animals, which repaired common deregulations in the production of metabolism-regulating adipokines to encourage weight loss and stop the promotion of weight gain. The ability of polyphenols to provide this benefit was discussed in in chapter 5.

In 2007, researchers in Japan discovered a novel chemical in acerola fruit that they named aceronidin. Their research reported that aceronidin had very strong antioxidant actions as well as the ability to block sugars from being absorbed by inhibiting a digestive enzyme, alpha-glucosidase, as well as the alpha-amylase enzyme that breaks down starches into sugars.

The anti-obesity research on acerola thus far confirms thousands of other independent studies by many that report antioxidants are helpful to prevent obesity as well as treat it. Reducing our ROS levels reduces all the damage ROS causes that promotes weight gain. The ability of acerola to interfere with sugar and starch absorption, thereby reducing the amount of calories absorbed during high-sugar and high-starch meals, is just more good news that acerola can help people lose weight.

Better Memory and Brain Function

As discussed earlier, free radicals and the damage they cause are implicated as a cause or significant cofactor in the development and progression of memory and brain disorders. You also learned that vitamin and polyphenol antioxidants are important natural substances that can treat and prevent these problems. During the electron transfer in the respiratory chain (how we metabolize the oxygen we breathe), free radicals are produced, which may damage the mitochondrial respiratory chain if our built-in antioxidant system is faltering. The brain is particularly vulnerable to the production of ROS because it metabolizes 20 percent of the total body oxygen and has a limited antioxidant capacity. Brain cells just don't store as much or as many of the natural antioxidants we produce in other cells in our bodies to reduce ROS naturally. That makes polyphenols and plant antioxidants important to support healthy brain function to pick up the slack.

There are countless studies published about polyphenols preventing or treating dementia, Alzheimer's disease, Parkinson's disease, and other brain disorders by reducing ROS and the oxidative stress, cellular damage, cell death, and chronic inflammation caused by excess ROS in the brain. Many other studies report these natural antioxidants can also increase memory through the same mechanisms of actions. With acerola providing one of the highest antioxidant potentials in natural plants, it's not unusual that scientists would study its effect on brain function.

In addition to the study reporting brain cell improvements for weight loss discussed in the previous section, another research group reported in 2018 that acerola juice protected the brain cells of adult and aged rats from chemicals meant to replicate aging in the brain, in addition to repairing aged brain cells in older rats. The hippocampus in the brain is largely responsible for memory and accumulation of free radicals, and the damage they cause in the hippocampus is linked with age-related memory loss and dementia. Taking multiple strong antioxidants, like those found in acerola, supports better brain function, including better memory, as well as prevents neurodegenerative diseases as detailed in earlier chapters for polyphenol and vitamin C actions and benefits.

Anti-Fatigue Actions

One of the easiest ways to maintain good energy levels (besides getting enough sleep) is to keep free radicals in check with a healthy and high-functioning natural antioxidant system. Oxidative stress can impact energy levels on a cellular level in numerous ways. Oxidative stress in the mitochondria of many cell types can lower the cellular energy these cells need to do their jobs, and this alone can contribute to both mental and physical fatigue. For example, when muscle cells don't have enough cellular energy, it causes weak muscles that tire out more easily. When mitochondrial dysfunction from free radicals is affecting the cardiovascular system, then less oxygen is carried through the bloodstream to all our cells, including the lungs, and we get winded and tire out more easily when we're physically active. Acerola's many natural antioxidants supporting our built-in antioxidant system to function at optimal levels is thought to significantly contribute to acerola's anti-fatigue benefits.

Many studies have been published on the anti-fatigue action of polyphenols in general, especially as it relates to exercise. When muscles are worked out strenuously, free radicals are generated as muscles are called on to metabolize more oxygen and glucose into cellular energy to perform harder or longer. Over 1,000 studies report that antioxidant supplementation of some sort benefits athletes and others performing strenuous exercise by more efficiently reducing these free radicals as they are formed, with an end result of more stamina and endurance and less pain and fatigue.

The anti-fatigue action of acerola was evaluated in 2018 by using a standard weight load swim test on trained mice. However, instead of using acerola fruit with all its natural antioxidant compounds, they extracted the pectin from acerola (acerola is about 4.5 percent pectin) and administered that to the animals instead. Acerola pectin had already been confirmed with strong antioxidant actions, among others. Researchers reported that acerola pectin at all dosages given reduced fatigue and allowed mice to swim farther and longer before exhaustion. It also improved all oxidative stress parameters they measured in muscles and in the brain, and it improved mitochondrial functions in both brain and muscle cells as well. Since the measured reduction of oxidative stress and better mitochondrial function was increased significantly in the hippocampus part of the brain in this research, this is further validation of the possibility of better memory, which was previously discussed.

Cancer Prevention and Anticancer Actions

It is well established that free radicals can damage DNA in various cells in our bodies. This DNA damage can result in a healthy cell mutating into a cancerous cell. For that reason, one of the main roles our natural built-in antioxidant system plays is to protect us from cancer by preventing the DNA damage free radicals can cause. This aspect is certainly a good reason to keep our antioxidant systems in good working order! Many plant polyphenol antioxidants, including those found in acerola, have been reported to protect cells from mutating into cancerous cells, and some have even been documented with the ability to repair the DNA damage caused by free radicals. This has resulted in many studies around the world reporting that polyphenol-rich diets and as well as supplements rich in polyphenols provide cancer-preventative actions. Acerola, with its high natural antioxidant levels, is no exception.

Acerola was first reported with anticancer actions by researchers in Japan in 2002. Their research suggested that pretreating mice with acerola protected them from developing induced lung cancer tumors by regulating abnormal cell growth at the initiation phase. This was probably the result of acerola's natural antioxidant compound's antimutagenic actions—it stopped the healthy cells from mutating into cancer cells. Researchers in Brazil also reported the antimutagenic action of acerola when they administered acerola to rats along with a chemotherapy drug (cyclophosphamide), which is known to cause oxidative and DNA damage to healthy cells. They reported in 2016 that the acerola was able to significantly reduce (by 80 to 90 percent) the amount of DNA damage caused by the drug when acerola was given to the animals as a pretreatment, in conjunction with and even after the chemo drug was administered.

Another research group in Japan tested acerola against several types oral cancers *in vitro* in 2004, including some multidrug-resistant strains. They reported that acerola was able to kill these cancer cells directly and reverse their drug resistance, without employing any antioxidant action. Since this study was only conducted in a test tube, much more research is required to confirm this ability in animals and humans. For this reason, there isn't enough research performed that acerola can actually treat cancer or kill cancer cells in the human body, and acerola shouldn't be promoted as such.

It is well established, however, that people who are battling cancer have a decreased antioxidant capacity, higher levels of damaging free radicals, and can be vitamin C deficient since their body's natural processes are trying to battle the cancer and are depleting these natural resources. These issues can be much worse while taking chemotherapy drugs. Taking acerola as nutritional support while battling cancer can be a good strategy.

Acerola's main role for cancer is in prevention. Supporting our natural antioxidant system, as described in this book, will provide benefits to protect healthy cells from turning into cancer cells. This is well established by a significant body of research.

Antidiabetic Actions

All the previously discussed AGE-inhibitor and cellular-protective antioxidant abilities of acerola holds important information for people with diabetes. Diabetes causes a significant amount of additional ROS and AGEs in numerous ways, which results in a chronic state of inflammation and oxidative stress.

It is well documented in thousands of studies that oxidative stress, chronic inflammation, and the resulting cellular damage caused by ROS and AGEs are a significant cause or cofactor of most diabetic complications, such as cardiovascular diseases, kidney damage resulting in renal failure, liver damage and fatty liver, nerve damage resulting in diabetic neuropathy, and macular degeneration. For these reasons, everyone with diabetes should consider eating an antioxidant-rich diet (lots of fresh vegetables and fruits) and taking strong cellular-protective antioxidant supplements like acerola if they want to avoid diabetic complications and co-occurring diseases.

Cellular-protective antioxidants and AGE inhibitors like those found in acerola may allow people with diabetes to live longer and manage their diabetes much more easily by avoiding many of these debilitating diabetic complications by effectively reducing ROS and AGEs, and the chronic inflammation and oxidative stress they cause.

Four studies have been published on acerola's benefits for diabetes, but they pertain to a completely different action—the ability of acerola to lower blood glucose levels or prevent them from rising. As discussed in the earlier section "Anti-Obesity and Weight-Loss Actions," acerola has been shown in research to inhibit the digestive enzymes that break down sugars during digestion (alpha-glucosidase) as well as the enzyme that breaks down starches into sugar molecules during digestion (alpha-amylase). If these sugar molecules are not broken down into smaller molecules that allow them to be absorbed by the body as glucose, then they are prevented from going into the bloodstream to raise blood glucose levels. Most of the antidiabetic animal research on acerola reports that administering acerola with high-sugar diets, or while loading animals with extra sugar, prevented blood sugar levels of the animals from rising as they normally should. The enzyme inhibition effects noted were stronger for alpha-glucosidase.

Generally, for this particular action to provide a benefit for diabetics, acerola should be taken if a high-sugar meal or snack is consumed. These digestive enzymes are released to digest food when we eat, and if the compounds in acerola can bind with these enzymes and interfere with their function, then the acerola needs to be present when these digestive enzymes go to work. These actions have not been studied in humans yet, so it's still unclear what specific benefits, and to what degree, acerola may provide for diabetics in this regard.

Antimicrobial Actions

Since polyphenols effectively protect plants from various bacteria, fungus, mold, and viruses, it's not unusual that a high-polyphenol fruit like acerola has been documented with the ability to kill or prevent the growth of these same disease-causing microorganisms. Acerola was first confirmed with the ability to kill fungi in 1993, and its ability to kill gram-positive bacteria like *Streptococcus* in 2004. The Japanese researchers publishing the 2004 study reported that acerola was ineffective against gram-negative bacterial strains like *E. coli* but highly effective in very low concentrations against the gram-positive bacteria they tested. A Brazilian researcher who has studied acerola extensively and published several studies on acerola's actions reported in several studies that acerola has good antibacterial actions against another gram-positive bacteria, *Staphylococcus aureus*.

A research group in Spain evaluated acerola's inhibitory activity against several meat spoilage bacteria and published their study in 2016. They focused on several strains of gram-negative *Pseudomonas* bacteria. These bacteria are considered the main contaminant bacteria of fresh meats stored under refrigeration and responsible for causing an off-odor and meat spoilage. Their *in vitro* tests of acerola indicated that it was highly active against all strains tested in very low concentrations. When they treated buffalo steaks in a water extract containing 8 percent acerola, they demonstrated that the treatment had a strong inhibition of both intentionally inoculated bacteria and naturally occurring microorganisms. Positive results, in terms of color and odor, were also observed during the entire storage of steaks preserved with the extract, which was related to acerola's antioxidant actions. Other researchers in Spain published a similar study in 2019 using acerola as an effective antimicrobial and antioxidant (natural preservative) additive ingredient for Spanish chorizo sausage. The antioxidant action of vitamin C as a natural food preservative is well established, so it's not surprising that a fruit high in vitamin C like acerola has this action as well.

Interestingly, a Brazilian university research group reported in 2017 that acerola's ability to prevent the growth of food-spoilage bacteria was by inhibiting bacterial communication known as quorum sensing. Researchers at the university have also recently started studying the antifungal actions of the acerola tree's leaves and published their first study in 2019.

Cholesterol-Lowering Actions

Many natural plant polyphenols have shown to be capable of affecting cholesterol levels in a great deal of research over the years. Another book in my Rainforest Medicinal

Plant Guide Series, *Hibiscus Flower: Nature's Secret for a Healthy Heart*, covers this topic extensively since human studies confirmed this plant's ability to lower cholesterol effectively. Hibiscus flowers and acerola share some of the same active polyphenol compounds that are providing these benefits; however, hibiscus contains a great deal more of these compounds than acerola delivers. Nevertheless, research has reported that acerola has these actions as well. Researchers at a university medical school in Brazil reported in 2011 that when acerola fruit was given to rats, it significantly lowered blood glucose and total cholesterol and triglycerides, but increased HDL cholesterol (the "good" cholesterol). Another Brazilian university research group confirmed these actions in 2018. Their study reported that giving acerola to rats fed a high-fat diet prevented cholesterol levels from rising, and it also promoted weight loss. They assumed these effects to be attributed to the polyphenol content of the acerola they gave the animals.

However, other research reports that, during human digestion, pectin binds to cholesterol in the gastrointestinal tract and slows the absorption of it by trapping carbohydrates. This ability may be playing a role in more healthful cholesterol levels since both plants contain a significant amount of natural pectin (but again, acerola's pectin content is less than hibiscus flower's).

After reading the research on polyphenols and cholesterol and the actual research on both rainforest plants, I believe that acerola's action in this regard to be a possible beneficial "side effect" that may occur when taking acerola for other health or wellness reasons. Based on the research, I will still continue to rely on hibiscus flowers instead of acerola to actually treat high cholesterol and the many problems that causes in the cardiovascular system.

Benefits for the Skin

As discussed earlier, acerola contains natural compounds that inhibit the production and damage of advanced glycation end products (AGEs). These AGEs accumulate in our skin cells over time and cause wrinkles, drier skin, and skin fragility as we age. AGEs also cause "browning" of the cells they glycate, so they are implicated in development of age spots (spots on the skin that are dark brown in color) that develop on our skin as we age. You also learned in that section that vitamin C plays an essential role in making new collagen that our skin needs for a youthful appearance. Free radicals also promote oxidative stress in the mitochondria of skin cells, which slow down normal functions (including the ability of skin cells to make collagen) and ages skin cells. Therefore, when we take acerola internally, we are interrupting several processes that can age our skin prematurely with acerola's antioxidant and AGE-inhibitor polyphenol and vitamin compounds. This can nutritionally support the skin and promote a more youthful appearance. And who doesn't want that?

Acerola may also provide these benefits when it is applied directly to the skin through similar actions. It is starting to show up in various skin-care and antiwrinkle cream products more regularly for these reasons. In addition, acerola contains several mineral salts that have shown to aid in the remineralization of tired and stressed skin, and its mucilage and proteins have skin-hydrating properties and promote capillary conditioning. Other antioxidants in acerola have been reported in research to brighten the skin and block harmful UV radiation. Three studies on these actions and benefits have been published between 2008 and 2017.

The first study was conducted in China in 2008 and used guinea pigs to determine if taking acerola orally would have an effect on the skin. They reported that administering a crude polyphenol extract of acerola orally protected the animals' skin, which had been subjected to controlled UVB irradiation and prevented it from browning (tanning). They attributed acerola's skin-lightening effect to the anthocyanin polyphenols in the acerola extract they gave the animals. The second study was conducted at the University Florida, which evaluated the *in vitro* action of various natural oils and fruit extracts, including acerola, to be applied topically to the skin and compared that to the actions of commercial sunscreen products. While they noted that the fruit extracts tested did provide sunscreen actions (and much better than the oils tested), the action was less than what commercial UV-blocking sunscreens provide.

The most recent study was conducted in Japan and published in 2017. They used a special species of hairless mice and gave them acerola juice to drink while they were being exposed to UVB irradiation over six weeks. Like the first study, they also reported that consumption of acerola juice was effective in suppressing UVB-induced skin pigmentation. Melanin is the main pigment in our skin cells that causes browning or the ability to tan skin, and it is produced in skin cells through a multistage chemical process known as melanogenesis. Both of these studies surmised that acerola's main mechanism of action was to inhibit melanogenesis.

It has been well documented by research that excessive sun damage to the skin promotes the production of free radicals, which damages these cells on a cellular level, and the DNA damage caused by free radicals can mutate normal skin cells into cancerous cells. Natural antioxidants applied topically and taken internally can be beneficial to counteract this process.

Summary

That a single exotic tropical fruit can provide so many different benefits is pretty amazing. This book began by asking, "What if there were just one supplement you could take that would make you look and feel younger, help you lose weight, give you more energy, make you smarter, and decrease your risk of developing a host of chronic diseases?" I hope that after reading this chapter, you understand why and how acerola can deliver these types of benefits. Acerola has been marketed and sold for far too many years as just a natural vitamin C supplement, which has greatly undervalued its true benefits. This book provides the information consumers need to determine acerola's far-reaching benefits.

CHAPTER 8

A Consumer Guide
for Acerola

A cerola supplements have been available for years and marketed as a vitamin C supplement. Once consumers learn of acerola's many other benefits as outlined in this book, the demand and use of acerola will increase.

Traditional Preparation

The traditional preparation of acerola is simply eating this tropical fruit as a healthy food in the tropics where it grows. Acerola fruit juices are bottled and consumed frequently in tropical countries that grow it. Acerola fruit is highly perishable so exports of the fresh fruit into the United States are not feasible.

The Safety of Acerola

The very long history of use of acerola as a food has established that this natural tropical fruit is safe and well tolerated with few, if any, side effects. Acerola has been added to commercially produced baby foods and fruit juice blends since the 1950s to increase the vitamin C content in these foods and beverages. Acerola has GRAS status (Generally Regarded as Safe) as a food additive from the Food and Drug Administration (FDA). Several toxicity studies, which are listed in the references section, have been performed in animals. Acerola, with its natural vitamin C, has not been documented with any side effects in the research studies published to date. However, high dosages (over 4 grams) of synthetic vitamin C (ascorbic acid) are associated with side effects, including stomach pain/cramps, diarrhea, nausea/vomiting, appetite loss, increased sweating, increased swelling, and abdominal pain.

Contraindications

❏ A study published in 2002 reported that acerola caused allergic reactivity similar to that of the well-known allergen latex. Those who may be allergic to latex may also be allergic to acerola in supplement form or to its addition in various fruit juices. Although this was a single isolated report, if you have a latex allergy, it's better to err on the side of caution and avoid using acerola.

❏ Large dosages (4 or more grams) of acerola may cause diarrhea.

Drug Interactions

❏ None reported.

Sources of Acerola

Most of the acerola sold in the United States has been plantation-grown in Brazil—the world's largest supplier (and consumer) of acerola products. Brazil currently has more than 25,000 acres under cultivation with acerola, which produces more than 30,000 metric tons of the fruit annually. About 60 percent is consumed locally with the remainder exported, mainly to the United States, Germany, France, and Japan.

Finding a Good Acerola Product

First, look for a certified organic source of acerola. Other countries like Brazil have different regulations about pesticides that may be allowed in food crops that may be banned in the United States. More than 20 acerola organic growers have been registered as exporters of acerola products to the United States, so they aren't hard to find.

Freeze-Dried versus Spray-Dried

By far, the best product available is an unripe or partially ripe freeze-dried acerola product. These contain all the vital nutrients and polyphenols contained in the plant, along with its beneficial fiber and pectin, with just the large amount of water (up to 90 percent) removed by freeze-drying. This is the closest you can come to just eating the fresh fruit since fresh acerola is not available here, unless you live in the Southern United States and can grow it in a frost-free climate. And, remember, the vitamins and polyphenols are much higher in unripe fruit than ripe fruit. These products are available in bulk powders sold by the ounce or pound and can be found in some encapsulated products. The powders should be a light tan to light brown in color, rather than red or pink. Ripe fruit powders will be light red to light pink in color and will not contain as many nutrients and polyphenols. These powders are intended to be stirred into water, juice, or smoothies and measured by the teaspoonful. The taste of these unripe powers are rather bland other than just the tartness (which comes from the high vitamin C content). Only when acerola ripens does it develop its crisp apple flavor.

If you are looking for an acerola product in capsules or tablets, make sure to read the label closely and make sure it says "acerola fruit" and doesn't use the words "juice" or "extract" in the "Supplements Facts" panel. Also expect to see additives or flow agents as added ingredients on the label. The freeze-dried powder is difficult to encapsulate because it's a bit sticky, and flow agents are required to get in into a capsule.

The significant problem with buying a juice product, whether it's sold as a "acerola concentrated 4:1 extract" or a "acerola standardized extract" is that the manufacturing process left most of the beneficial polyphenols behind. Extract manufactures have concentrated on just extracting this fruit for its vitamin C for too many years and have long ignored the other beneficial plant compound that acerola provides.

The most prevalent (and cheapest) product sold today is a spray-dried juice powder which I don't recommend. To make this product, acerola fruit is chopped up, added to water, and juiced (by mechanically squeezing or pressing). The juice is then mixed with sugar: typically 50 percent juice to 50 percent corn sugar (maltodextrin), and then another 5 to 15 percent of maltodextrin dextrose (more sugar) is added in. This is then sprayed on a hot rotating barrel that quickly evaporates off the water/moisture at very high temperature until only a powder remains. By volume, it can be 75 percent or more corn sugar, but it is soluble in water and is easy to make capsule and tablet products with.

But the real problem is that most of the polyphenols have been left behind with the leftover pulp and skins after juicing. All "the stuff" left over after juicing a fruit is called "bagasse" in Brazil. Other countries typically call it agro-industrial waste since it has to be disposed of after the fruit is processed into juice. Brazilian juice manufacturers have discovered the polyphenol problem in their juices, but instead of changing methods to get more polyphenols into their juice, they now just use the terminology of "byproduct" instead of bagasse. Turn to "Processing and Manufacturing Methods" in the references section to see the studies published on acerola's bagasse, or byproduct, and why the industry is researching how they can either "re-extract" the bagasse utilizing a different method, or simply dry out the bagasse and grind it into a "flour" or powder to sell again as a polyphenol-rich acerola "byproduct." You'll also find a listing of independent studies comparing the nutrients and polyphenols in spray-dried and freeze-dried acerola that researchers tested.

Since the "leftover stuff" after juicing acerola (around 40 percent of the fruit volume) is so rich in beneficial polyphenols, one has to wonder just how many of these beneficial compounds actually got squeezed out into the juice! One of these studies evaluating the byproduct reported that there were much more anthocyanins and flavonoids (the main polyphenols in acerola) in the byproduct than were in the juice. Unfortunately, this is never evaluated or enumerated by manufacturers selling acerola 4:1 juice extracts or standardized extracts since these products were manufactured and standardized to the vitamin C, not polyphenols or other nutrients.

That brings us to the final issue with the problems of these manufactured extracts. A great deal of the vitamin C can be lost in the high-heat, spray-dry process utilized for acerola extracts, and even more is left behind in the byproduct after juicing. Some manufacturers are willing and capable of just adding cheap synthetic ascorbic acid to their extract products to replace the natural vitamin C that was lost by their processing. This has also been an issue with the so-called standardized extracts of acerola that are guaranteed to contain a specific amount of vitamin C. Some manufacturers of these products just add synthetic ascorbic acid to meet the promised amount of vitamin C rather than using more fruit to further concentrate acerola to provide the natural version. In the U.S. acerola import market, the most common adulterant affecting product quality is synthetic ascorbic acid, and for that reason, a special test was devised to counteract this problem.

This brings us to the final point: if you want to find a good acerola product and/or if you choose an extract product, you need to choose a good reputable U.S. manufacturer. Ethical manufacturers have a laboratory test they can use (if they choose to) that will determine if synthetic ascorbic acid is adulterating the acerola extract they purchase to make their products.

With all these inherent issues with acerola extracts, my personal choice is to stick with a natural freeze-dried acerola product and know that I'm getting all the natural compounds that were tested in this beneficial nutrient-dense tropical fruit without any human interference (and without all that added sugar). I also know that I have to pay more money for freeze-dried products, but at least I know what I am getting.

Where to Purchase Acerola

Acerola products are sold under various brand names and are widely available in health food stores and through online retailers. The acerola name is the official accepted common name in the U.S. market, so product labels can just use this name without displaying the scientific name on a label. If the scientific name is used on a label, it can be one of the three names mentioned in chapter 1: *Malpighia glabra*, *Malpighia emarginata*, or *Malpighia punicifolia*. Acerola can also be found as an ingredient in various dietary supplements, including multivitamins, as well as in various body-care products and face creams. Acerola's status as a "superfruit" has been well established in the marketplace, and it is showing up in a growing number of functional foods and beverages in the natural products market.

Suggested Dosages Acerola

Oftentimes, the dosages used and recommended for acerola follow the dosages used for vitamin C. The adult recommended dietary allowance (RDA) for vitamin C is 60 to 75 milligrams daily. However, most of the research reporting therapeutic benefits were using, on average, 1 gram (1,000 milligrams) daily in their studies. Therapeutic dosages of vitamin C for colds and flu, general illnesses, and debility are 1 to 5 grams daily. The average freeze-dried acerola powder contains around 750 to 1,000 milligrams of vitamin C per teaspoon of powder.

For general prevention and to support your built-in antioxidant system, use 1 teaspoon of a freeze-dried acerola powder daily stirred into water, juice, a cup of hot tea, or blended into a smoothie. It can even be sprinkled over salads or other foods as you'd use lemon juice for flavoring. This amount is comparable to the dosages in the research on acerola to address common free radical issues. If you want to try acerola for weight loss, take 1 teaspoon of the freeze-dried powder 10 minutes before each meal with 8 ounces of water.

Therapeutic dosages in times of stress and illness, or if you have a diet or lifestyle that promotes more free radicals, use 1 teaspoon of the freeze-dried powder two or three times daily. You can substitute capsules for the powder if you prefer; just determine how many capsules are required to equal these recommended amounts (capsules sizes can vary).

If you have a cold, flu, sore throat, or strep throat, dissolve 1 teaspoon of the powder in an 8-ounce cup of warm water, add the juice of half a lemon, and 3 tablespoons of raw honey and sip slowly. Repeat several times daily.

Conclusion

The recent growth in the knowledge of free radicals and the many diseases they can cause is producing a medical revolution that promises a new age of health and disease management. Acerola's ability to fight free radicals more effectively than natural products and foods puts acerola in the front line for this revolution. While vitamin C is one of the more important antioxidants that our bodies need to fight free radicals, and acerola delivers an astounding amount of vitamin C, acerola is more than just this one important nutrient.

Tens of thousands of research studies have been published in just the last five years on the actions and benefits of antioxidant polyphenols and their benefits to treat and prevent numerous diseases and conditions. If you choose a good acerola product using the information provided in this book, your ability to support your in-house antioxidant system with a significant amount of beneficial polyphenols combined with vitamin C may well be what's missing in your diet that is putting you at risk for developing many chronic diseases.

While eating healthy, maintaining a healthy weight, and avoiding bad habits like smoking are the best road to health and wellness through lowering free radicals in our bodies, the sad fact is most of us don't always achieve that, at least not all the time. Our current diets and hurried, and stressful lifestyles are bombarding our bodies with free radicals—there will be an eventual price to pay. This can be clearly seen in the rising rates of obesity, heart disease, type 2 diabetes, Alzheimer's disease, and other chronic diseases we're seeing today.

Acerola is *not* the answer to all disease or some cure-all panacea; it is simply an effective tool to be used to help your body fight free radicals and to help keep your own defensive antioxidant system healthy and performing the important job it was designed to do.

References

This reference list was complete the day it was compiled; however, new studies are frequently published on this important medicinal plant. The citations below are listed in chronological order with the newest research listed first. Visit www.pubmed.gov to access the latest studies cataloged at the U.S. National Library of Medicine (PubMed). More information and periodic updated references on the research on acerola can be found in the Rain-Tree Tropical Plant Database file for acerola online at http://rain-tree.com/acerola.htm.

Chapter 1. What Is Acerola?

Asenjo, C. and Freire, D. "The high ascorbic acid content of the West Indian cherry." *Science*. 1946; 103(2669): 219.

Assis, S., et al. "Acerola: importance, culture conditions, production and biochemical aspects." *Fruits*. 2008; 63(2): 93–101.

Badejo, A., et al. "Cloning and expression of GDP-D-mannose pyrophosphorylase gene and ascorbic acid content of acerola (*Malpighia glabra* L.) fruit at ripening stages." *Plant. Physiol. Biochem.* 2007 Sep; 45(9): 665–72.

Derse, P., "Nutrient content of acerola, a rich source of vitamin C." *J. Am. Med. Assoc.* 1954 Dec 18; 156(16): 1501.

de Medeiros, R. "Proportion of ascorbic, dehydroascorbic and diketogulonic acids in green or ripe acerola (*Malpighia punicifolia*)." *Rev. Bras. Med.* 1969 Jul; 26(7): 398–400.

Floch, H., et al. "West Indian cherry, *Malpighia punicifolia* L., its exceptional richness in vitamin C." *Publ. Inst. Pasteur Guyane. Fr. Inini.* 1955 Jul; 16 (368): 1–6.

Hanamura, T., et al. "Changes of the composition in acerola (*Malpighia emarginata* DC.) fruit in relation to cultivar, growing region and maturity." *J. Sci. Food Ag.* 2008 Aug; 88(10): 1813–1820.

Lima, V., et al. "Total phenolic and carotenoid contents in acerola genotypes harvested at three ripening stages." *Food Chem.* 2005 May; 90(4): 565–568.

Mustard, M. "The ascorbic acid content of some *Malpighia* fruits and jellies." *Science.* 1946 Sep; 104(2697): 230.

Chapter 2. Free Radicals and Antioxidants

Aruoma, O., et al. "Nutrition and health aspects of free radicals and antioxidants." *Food Chem. Toxicol.* 1994; 32: 671–83.

Bagchi, K., and Puri, S. "Free radicals and antioxidants in health and disease." *East Mediterranean Health J.* 1998; 4: 350–60.

Cheeseman, K., et al. "An introduction to free radical biochemistry." *Br. Med. Bull.* 1993 Jul; 49(3): 481–93.

Halliwell, B. and Gutteridge, J. "*Free radicals in biology and medicine.*" 4th ed. Oxford, UK: Clarendon Press; 2007.

Housset, B. "Biochemical aspects of free radicals metabolism." *Bull. Eur. Physiopathol. Respir.* 1987 Jul–Aug; 23(4): 287–90.

Lobo, V., et al. "Free radicals, antioxidants and functional foods: Impact on human health." *Pharmacogn. Rev.* 2010 Jul–Dec; 4(8): 118–126.

Matsuda, M., et al. "Increased oxidative stress in obesity: implications for metabolic syndrome, diabetes, hypertension, dyslipidemia, atherosclerosis, and cancer." *Obes. Res. Clin. Pract.* 2013; 7: e330–e341.

Pham-Huv, L., et al. "Free radicals, antioxidants in disease and health." *Int. J. Biomed. Sci.* 2008 Jun; 4(2): 89–96.

Rock, C., "Update on biological characteristics of the antioxidant micronutrients –Vitamin C, Vitamin E and the carotenoids." *J. Am. Diet. Assoc.* 1996; 96: 693–702.

Sagnoun, Z., et al. "Free radicals and antioxidants: human physiology, pathology and therapeutic aspects." *Therapie.* 1997 Jul–Aug; 52(4):251–70.

Valko, M., et al. "Free radicals and antioxidants in normal physiological functions and human disease." *Review. Int. J. Biochem. Cell Biol.* 2007; 39: 44–84.

Xu, D., et al. "Natural antioxidants in foods and medicinal plants: extraction, assessment and resources." *Int. J. Mol. Sci.* 2017 Jan; 18(1): 96.

Young, I. and Woodside, J. "Antioxidants in health and disease." *J. Clin. Pathol.* 2001; 54: 176–186.

Chapter 3. The Health Benefits of Vitamin C

Ali, S., et al. "Understanding oxidants and antioxidants: Classical team with new players." *J. Food Biochem.* 2020 Jan; 13145. (ahead of print)

Amr, M., et al. "Efficacy of vitamin C as an adjunct to fluoxetine therapy in pediatric major depressive disorder: A randomized, double-blind, placebo-controlled pilot study." *Nutr. J.* 2013; 12: 31.

Ashor, A., et al. "Effect of vitamin C on endothelial function in health and disease: a systematic review and meta-analysis of randomised controlled trials." *Atherosclerosis.* 2014 Jul; 235(1): 9–20.

Baxter, R., et al. "Vitamin C and glaucoma." *J. Am. Optom. Assoc.* 1988 Jun; 59(6): 438.

Bowers, E., et al. "Vitamin C levels in old people and the response to ascorbic acid and to the juice of the acerola (*Malpighia punicifolia* L.)." *Br. J. Clin. Pract.* 1965 Mar; 19: 141–7.

Carr, A. and Maggini, S. "Vitamin C and immune function." *Nutrients.* 2017 Nov; 9(11): E1211.

Carr, A., "Synthetic or food-derived vitamin C - are they equally bioavailable?" *Nutrients.* 2013 Nov; 5(11): 4284–4304.

Chen, K., et al. "Vitamin C suppresses oxidative lipid damage *in vivo*, even in the presence of iron overload." *Am. J. Physiol. Endocrinol. Metab.* 2000; 279: E1406-12.

Choi, H., et al. "Vitamin C intake and the risk of gout in men: a prospective study." *Arch. Intern. Med.* 2009 Mar; 169(5): 502–7.

Clein, N., "Acerola juice, the richest known source of vitamin C; A clinical study in infants." *J. Pediatr.* 1956 Feb; 48(2): 140–5.

Colagar, A., et al. "Ascorbic acid in human seminal plasma: determination and its relationship to sperm quality." *J. Clin. Biochem. Nutr.* 2009 Sep; 45(2): 144–9.

Cosgrove, M., et al. "Dietary nutrient intakes and skin-aging appearance among middle-aged American women." *Am. J. Clin. Nutr.* 2007; 86: 1225–1231.

de Oliveira, I., et al. "Effects of oral vitamin C supplementation on anxiety in students: a double-blind, randomized, placebo-controlled trial." *Pak. J. Biol. Sci.* 2015 Jan; 18(1): 11–8.

Fidanza, A., et al. "Therapeutic action of vitamin C on cholesterol metabolism." *Boll. Soc. Ital. Biol. Sper.* 1979 Mar; 55(6): 553–8.

Fiorani, M., et al. "Mitochondrial reactive oxygen species: The effects of mitochondrial ascorbic acid vs untargeted and mitochondria-targeted antioxidants." *Int. J. Radiat. Biol.* 2020 Jan 24: 1–25.

Gale, C., et al. "Cognitive impairment and mortality in a cohort of elderly people." *BMJ.* 1996 Mar; 312(7031): 608–11.

Gautam, M., et al. "Role of antioxidants in generalised anxiety disorder and depression." *Indian J. Psychiatry.* 2012; 54: 244–247.

Goodwin, J., et al. "Association between nutritional status and cognitive functioning in a healthy elderly population." *JAMA.* 1983 Jun; 249(21): 2917–21.

Hagel, A., et al. "Intravenous infusion of ascorbic acid decreases serum histamine concentrations in patients with allergic and non-allergic diseases." *Naunyn. Schmiedebergs Arch. Pharmacol.* 2013 Sep; 386(9): 789–93.

Hemila, H. "Vitamin C and common cold-induced asthma: a systematic review and statistical analysis." *Allergy Asthma Clin. Immunol.* 2013 Nov; 9(1): 46.

Hemila, H., et al. "Vitamin C for preventing and treating the common cold." *Cochrane Database Syst Rev.* 2013 Jan 31; (1): CD000980.

Huijskens, M., et al. "Technical advance: ascorbic acid induces development of double-positive T cells from human hematopoietic stem cells in the absence of stromal cells." *J. Leukoc. Biol.* 2014 Dec; 96(6): 1165–75.

Hysi, P., et al. "Ascorbic acid metabolites are involved in intraocular pressure control in the general population." *Redox Biol.* 2019 Jan; 20: 349–353.

Johnston, C., et al. "Antihistamine effect of supplemental ascorbic acid and neutrophil chemotaxis." *J. Am. Coll. Nutr.* 1992 Apr; 11(2): 172–6.

Juraschek, S., et al. "Effect of oral vitamin C supplementation on serum uric acid: a meta-analysis of randomized controlled trials." *Arthritis Care Res.* 2011 Sep; 63(9): 1295–306.

Juraschek, S., et al. "Effects of vitamin C supplementation on blood pressure: a meta-analysis of randomized controlled trials." *Am. J. Clin. Nutr.* 2012 May; 95(5): 1079–88.

References

Kim, S., et al. "Consumption of high-dose vitamin C (1250 mg per day) enhances functional and structural properties of serum lipoprotein to improve anti-oxidant, anti-atherosclerotic, and anti-aging effects via regulation of anti-inflammatory microRNA." *Food Funct.* 2015 Nov; 6(11): 3604–12.

Knekt, P., et al. "Antioxidant vitamins and coronary heart disease risk: a pooled analysis of 9 cohorts." *Am. J. Clin. Nutr.* 2004 Dec; 80(6): 1508–20.

Kocot, J., et al. "Does vitamin C influence neurodegenerative diseases and psychiatric disorders?" *Nutrients.* 2017 Jun; 9(7): E659.

Kurti, S., et al. "Improved lung function following dietary antioxidant supplementation in exercise-induced asthmatics." *Respir. Physiol. Neurobiol.* 2016 Jan; 220: 95–101.

Luck, M., et al. "Ascorbic acid and fertility." *Biol. Reprod.* 1995 Feb; 52(2): 262–6.

Mao, X and Yao, G. "Effect of vitamin C supplementations on iron deficiency anemia in Chinese children." *Biomed. Environ. Sci.* 1992 Jun; 5(2): 125–9.

McArdle, F., et al. "UVR-induced oxidative stress in human skin *in vivo*: effects of oral vitamin C supplementation." *Free Radic. Biol. Med.* 2002; 33: 1355–1362.

McRae, M. "Vitamin C supplementation lowers serum low-density lipoprotein cholesterol and triglycerides: a meta-analysis of 13 randomized controlled trials." *J. Chiropr. Med.* 2008 Jun; 7(2): 48–58.

Mikirova, N., et al. "The effect of high dose IV vitamin C on plasma antioxidant capacity and level of oxidative stress in cancer patients and healthy subjects." *J. Orthomol. Med.* 2007; 22: 3.

Moser, M., et al. "Vitamin C and heart health: A review based on findings from epidemiologic studies." *Int. J. Mol. Sci.* 2016 Aug 12; 17(8).

Nauman, G., et al. "Systematic review of intravenous ascorbate in cancer clinical trials." *Antioxidants.* 2018 Jul; 7(7): E89.

Ngo, B., et al. "Targeting cancer vulnerabilities with high-dose vitamin C." 2019 Apr; 19: 271–282.

Padayatty, S., et al. "Vitamin C as an antioxidant: Evaluation of its role in disease prevention." *J. Am. Coll. Nutr.* 2003; 22: 18–35.

Paleologos, M., et al. "Cohort study of vitamin C intake and cognitive impairment." *Am. J. Epidemiol.* 1998 Jul; 148(1): 45–50.

Popovic, L., et al. "Influence of vitamin C supplementation on oxidative stress and neutrophil inflammatory response in acute and regular exercise." *Oxid. Med. Cell. Longev.* 2015 Feb; 2015: 295497.

Rafiee, B., et al. "Comparing the effectiveness of dietary vitamin C and exercise interventions on fertility parameters in normal obese men." *Urol. J.* 2016 Apr; 13(2): 2635–9.

Ramdas, W., et al. "The Effect of vitamins on glaucoma: A systematic review and meta-analysis." *Nutrients.* 2018 Mar; 10(3): E359.

Ran, L., et al. "Extra dose of vitamin C based on a daily supplementation shortens the common cold: a meta-analysis of 9 randomized controlled trials." *Biomed. Res. Int.* 2018 Jul; 2018: 1837634.

Retsky, K., et al. "Ascorbic acid oxidation product(s) protect human low density lipoprotein against atherogenic modification. Anti-rather than prooxidant activity of vitamin C in the presence of transition metal ions." *J. Biol. Chem.* 1993; 268: 1304–9.

Rubio-Lopez, N., et al. "Nutrient intake and depression symptoms in Spanish children: The ANIVA Study." *Int. J. Environ. Res. Public Health.* 2016; 13: 352.

Sanchez-Quesada, J., et al. "Ascorbic acid inhibits the increase in low-density lipoprotein (LDL) susceptibility to oxidation and the proportion of electronegative LDL induced by intense aerobic exercise." *Coron. Artery Dis.* 1998; 9(5): 249–55.

Schencking, M., et al. "Intravenous vitamin C in the treatment of shingles: results of a multicenter prospective cohort study." *Med. Sci. Monit.* 2012 Apr; 18(4): CR215–24.

Taddei, S., et al. "Vitamin C improves endothelium-dependent vasodilation by restoring nitric oxide activity in essential hypertension." *Circulation* 1998; 97: 2222–9.

Tang, L. "Comparative study of the bioavailability of ascorbic acid in commercially produced products." [Dissertation] 1995; University of Pennsylvania, Department of Chemistry.

Turley, S., et al. "The role of ascorbic acid in the regulation of cholesterol metabolism and in the pathogenesis of atherosclerosis." *Atherosclerosis.* 1976 Jul-Aug; 24(1-2): 1–18.

Uchida, E., et al. "Absorption and excretion of ascorbic acid alone and in acerola (*Malpighia emarginata*) juice: comparison in healthy Japanese subjects." *Biol. Pharm. Bull.* 2011; 34(11): 1744–7.

Volbracht, C., et al. "Intravenous vitamin C in the treatment of allergies: an interim subgroup analysis of a long-term observational study." *J. Int. Med. Res.* 2018 Sep; 46(9): 3640–3655.

Wang, K., et al. "Role of vitamin C in skin diseases." *Front. Physiol.* 2018 Jul; 9: 819.

Ye, Z., et al. "Antioxidant vitamins intake and the risk of coronary heart disease: meta-analysis of cohort studies." *Eur. J. Cardiovasc. Prev. Rehabil.* 2008 Feb;15(1): 26–34.

Zhang, M., et al. "Vitamin C provision improves mood in acutely hospitalized patients." *Nutrition.* 2011; 27: 530–533.

Chapter 4. The Power of Polyphenols

An, J., et al. "Natural products for treatment of osteoporosis: The effects and mechanisms on promoting osteoblast-mediated bone formation." *Life Sci.* 2016 Feb 15; 147: 46–58.

Ashok, B., et al. "The aging paradox: Free radical theory of aging." *Exp. Gerontol.* 1999; 34: 293–303.

Assini, E., et al. "Antiobesity effects of anthocyanins in preclinical and clinical studies." *Oxid. Med. Cell. Longev.* 2017; 2017: 2740364.

Bijak, M., et al. "Popular naturally occurring antioxidants as potential anticoagulant drugs." *Chem. Biol. Interact.* 2016 Sep; 257: 35–45.

Bijak, M., et al. "Polyphenol compounds belonging to flavonoids inhibit activity of coagulation factor X." *Int. J. Biol. Macromol.* 2014 Apr; 65: 129–35.

Callejo, M., et al. "Impact of nutrition on pulmonary arterial hypertension." *Nutrients.* 2020 Jan; 12(1): E169.

Carrasco-Pozo, C., et al. "Quercetin and epigallocatechin gallate in the prevention and treatment of obesity: from molecular to clinical studies." *J. Med. Food.* 2019 Aug; 22(8): 753–770.

Correa, T., et al. "The two-way polyphenols-microbiota interactions and their effects on obesity and related metabolic diseases." *Front. Nutr.* 2019 Dec; 6: 188.

Chen, Y., et al. "Polyphenols and oxidative stress in atherosclerosis-related ischemic heart disease and stroke." *Oxid. Med. Cell. Longev.* 2017; 2017: 8526438.

Davinelli, S., et al. "Cytoprotective polyphenols against chronological skin aging and cutaneous photodamage." *Curr. Pharm. Des.* 2018; 24(2): 99–105.

Dilberger, B., et al. "Polyphenols and metabolites enhance survival in rodents and nematodes-impact of mitochondria." *Nutrients*. 2019 Aug; 11(8): E1886.

Dryden, G., et al. "Polyphenols and gastrointestinal diseases." *Curr. Opin. Gastroenterol.* 2006 Mar; 22(2): 165–170.

Grosso, G., et al. "Dietary polyphenol intake and risk of type 2 diabetes in the Polish arm of the health, alcohol and psychosocial factors in eastern Europe (HAPIEE) study." *Br. J. Nutr.* 2017 Jul 14; 118(1): 60–68.

Hussain, T., et al. "Oxidative stress and inflammation: what polyphenols can do for us? *Oxid. Med. Cell. Longev.* 2016; 2016: 7432797.

Karim, N., et al. "An increasing role of polyphenols as novel therapeutics for Alzheimer's: A review." *Med. Chem.* 2019; Nov 5. (ahead of print)

Kim, Y., et al. "Polyphenols and glycemic control." *Nutrients*. 2016 Jan; 8(1): 17.

Li, A., et al. "Resources and biological activities of natural polyphenols." *Nutrients*. 2014 Dec; 6(12): 6020–6047.

Liu, J., et al. "Beneficial effects of dietary polyphenols on high-fat diet-induced obesity linking with modulation of gut microbiota." *J. Agric. Food Chem.* 2020 Jan; 68(1): 33–47.

Majidinia, M., et al. "Targeting miRNAs by polyphenols: Novel therapeutic strategy for aging." *Biochem. Pharmacol.* 2019 Nov 1: 113688. (ahead of print)

Marchesi, J., et al. "The gut microbiota and host health: a new clinical frontier." *Gut*. 2016 Feb; 65(2): 330–9.

Marin, L., et al. "Bioavailability of dietary polyphenols and gut microbiota metabolism: antimicrobial properties." *Biomed. Res. Int.* 2015; 2015: 905215.

Niedzwiecki, A., et al. "Anticancer efficacy of polyphenols and their combinations." *Nutrients*. 2016 Sep; 8(9): 552.

Pacheco-Ordaz, R., et al. "Effect of phenolic compounds on the growth of selected probiotic and pathogenic bacteria." *Lett. Appl. Microbiol.* 2018 Jan; 66(1): 25–31.

Poti, F., et al. "Polyphenol health effects on cardiovascular and neurodegenerative disorders: a review and meta-analysis." *Int. J. Mol. Sci.* 2019 Jan; 20(2): 351.

Ribeiro da Silva, L., et al. "Quantification of bioactive compounds in pulps and by-products of tropical fruits from Brazil." *Food Chem.* 2014 Jan; 143: 398–404.

References

Rienks, J., et al. "Association of polyphenol biomarkers with cardiovascular disease and mortality risk: A systematic review and meta-analysis of observational studies." *Nutrients.* 2017 Apr; 9(4): 415.

Righetto, A., et al. "Chemical composition and antioxidant activity of juices from mature and immature acerola (*Malpighia emarginata* DC)." 2005 Aug; 11(4): 315–321.

Rowland, I., et al. "Gut microbiota functions: metabolism of nutrients and other food components." *Eur. J. Nutr.* 2018 Feb; 57(1): 1–24.

Russo, G., et al. "Mechanisms of aging and potential role of selected polyphenols in extending healthspan." *Biochem. Pharmacol.* 2019 Nov 21: 113719.

Silva, R., et al. "Polyphenols from food and natural products: neuroprotection and safety." *Antioxidants.* 2020 Jan; 9(1): E61.

Silvester, A., et al. "Dietary polyphenols and their roles in fat browning." *J. Nutr. Biochem.* 2019 Feb; 64: 1–12.

Tangney, C., et al. "Polyphenols, inflammation, and cardiovascular disease." *Curr. Atheroscler. Rep.* 2013 May; 15(5): 324.

Vendramini, A., et al. "Phenolic compounds in acerola fruit (*Malpighia punicifolia,* L.)." *J. Braz. Chem. Soc.* 2004; 15(5): 664–668.

Williamson, G., et al. "The role of polyphenols in modern nutrition." *Nutr. Bull.* 2017 Sep; 42(3): 226–235.

Xiao, J., et al. "Dietary polyphenols and type 2 diabetes: current insights and future perspectives." *Curr. Med. Chem.* 2015; 22(1): 23–38.

Zang, H., et al. "Dietary polyphenols, oxidative stress and antioxidant and anti-inflammatory effects." *Curr. Opin. Food Sci.* 2016 Apr; 8: 33–42.

Zhou, Y., et al. "Natural polyphenols for prevention and treatment of cancer." *Nutrients.* 2016 Aug; 8(8): 515.

Chapter 5. How Polyphenols and Antioxidants Prevent Disease

Bungau, S., et al. "Health benefits of polyphenols and carotenoids in age-related eye diseases." *Oxid. Med. Cell. Longev.* 2019; 2019: 9783429.

Cao, H., et al. "Dietary polyphenols and type 2 diabetes: human study and clinical trial." *Crit. Rev. Food Sci. Nutr.* 2019; 59(20): 3371–3379.

Ceriello, A., et al. "Possible role of oxidative stress in the pathogenesis of hypertension." *Diabetes Care.* 2008 Feb; 31 Suppl 2: S181–4.

Cheng, Y., et al. "Polyphenols and oxidative stress in atherosclerosis-related ischemic heart disease and stroke." *Oxid. Med. Cell. Longev.* 2017; 2017: 8526438.

De Bruyne, T., et al. "Dietary polyphenols targeting arterial stiffness: interplay of contributing mechanisms and gut microbiome-related metabolism." *Nutrients.* 2019 Mar; 11(3): 578.

Dunmore, S., et al. "The role of adipokines in β-cell failure of type 2 diabetes." *J. Endocrinol.* 2013 Jan; 216(1): T37–45.

Ellulu, M., et al. "Obesity and inflammation: the linking mechanism and the complications." *Arch. Med. Sci.* 2017; 13(4): 851–863.

Engin, A., et al. "The pathogenesis of obesity-associated adipose tissue inflammation." *Adv. Exp. Med. Biol.* 2017; 960: 221–245.

Fernández-Sánchez, A., et al. "Inflammation, oxidative stress, and obesity." *Int. J. Mol. Sci.* 2011; 12(5): 3117–3132.

Figueira, I., et al. "Polyphenols beyond barriers: a glimpse into the brain." *Curr. Neuropharmacol.* 2017 May; 15(4): 562–594.

Grootaert, C., et al. "Cell systems to investigate the impact of polyphenols on cardiovascular health." *Nutrients.* 2015 Nov; 7(11): 9229–9255.

Hussain, T., et al. "Oxidative stress and inflammation: what polyphenols can do for us?" *Oxid. Med. Cell. Longev.* 2016; 2016: 7432797.

Jan, F., et al. "Mitochondria-centric review of polyphenol bioactivity in cancer models." *Antioxid. Redox. Signal.* 2018 Dec; 29(16): 1589–1611.

Kim, Y., et al. "Polyphenols and glycemic control." *Nutrients.* 2016 Jan; 8(1): 17.

Koch, W. "Dietary polyphenols—important non-nutrients in the prevention of chronic noncommunicable diseases. a systematic review." *Nutrients.* 2019 May; 11(5): 1039.

Li, S., et al. "The potential and action mechanism of polyphenols in the treatment of liver diseases." *Oxid. Med. Cell. Longev.* 2018; 2018: 8394818.

Liang, W., et al. "The potential of adipokines as biomarkers and therapeutic agents for vascular complications in type 2 diabetes mellitus." *Cytokine Grow. Fact. Rev.* 2019 Aug; 48: 32–39.

Matsuda M, et al. "Increased oxidative stress in obesity: implications for metabolic syndrome, diabetes, hypertension, dyslipidemia, atherosclerosis, and cancer." *Obes. Res. Clin. Pract.* 2013; 7: e330–e341.

Mattera, R., et al. "Effects of polyphenols on oxidative stress-mediated injury in cardiomyocytes." *Nutrients*. 2017 May; 9(5): 523.

Mihaylova, D., et al. "Polyphenols as suitable control for obesity and diabetes." *Open Biotech. J.* 2010 Sept; 12: 219–228.

Naoi, M., et al. "Mitochondria in neuroprotection by phytochemicals: bioactive polyphenols modulate mitochondrial apoptosis system, function and structure." *Int. J. Mol. Sci.* 2019 May; 20(10): 2451.

Pasinetti, G., et al. "The Role of the gut microbiota in the metabolism of polyphenols as characterized by gnotobiotic mice." *J. Alzheimers Dis.* 2018; 63(2): 409–421.

Rienks, J., et al. "Polyphenol exposure and risk of type 2 diabetes: dose-response meta-analyses and systematic review of prospective cohort studies." *Am. J. Clin. Nutr.* 2018; 108: 49–61.

Silveira, A., et al. "The action of polyphenols in *Diabetes mellitus* and Alzheimer's disease: a common agent for overlapping pathologies." *Curr. Neuropharmacol.* 2019 Jul; 17(7): 590–613.

Serino, A., and Salazar, G. "Protective role of polyphenols against vascular inflammation, aging and cardiovascular disease." *Nutrients*. 2018 Dec; 11(1): E53.

Tressera-Rimbau, A., et al. "Dietary polyphenols in the prevention of stroke." *Oxid. Med. Cell. Longev.* 2017; 2017: 7467962.

Vauzour, D., et al. "Polyphenols and human health: prevention of disease and mechanisms of action." *Nutrients*. 2010 Nov; 2(11): 1106–1131.

Wang, X., et al. "Flavonoid intake and risk of CVD: a systematic review and meta-analysis of prospective cohort studies." *Br. J. Nutr.* 2014 Jan; 111(1): 1–11.

Woo, C., et al. "Mitochondrial dysfunction in adipocytes as a primary cause of adipose tissue inflammation." *Diabetes Metab. J.* 2019 Jun; 43(3): 247256.

Yahfoufi, N., et al. "The immunomodulatory and anti-inflammatory role of polyphenols." *Nutrients*. 2018 Nov; 10(11): 1618.

Chapter 6. The Benefits of Acerola in Fighting Free Radicals

Ajiboy, E. "Lophirones B and C attenuate acetaminophen-induced liver damage in mice: studies on hepatic, oxidative stress and inflammatory biomarkers." *J. Biochem. Mol. Toxicol.* 2016; 30(10): 497–505.

Almeida, I., et al. "Cytotoxic and mutagenic effects of iodine-131 and radioprotection of acerola (*Malpighia glabra* L.) and beta-carotene *in vitro*." *Genet. Mol. Res.* 2013 Dec 10; 12(4): 6402–13.

Alvarez-Suarez, J., et al. "The protective effect of acerola (*Malpighia emarginata*) against oxidative damage in human dermal fibroblasts through the improvement of antioxidant enzyme activity and mitochondrial functionality." *Food Funct.* 2017 Sep; 8(9): 3250–3258.

Bhargava, P., et al. "Screening acerola (*Malpighia emarginata*) genotypes for protection against LPS-induced inflammation in macrophage cells and selectivity to cyclooxygenase-2 (COX-2) activity." *FASEB J.* 2016 Apr; 30(1 Supl): 1174.24.

Barros, B., et al. "Saline extract from *Malpighia emarginata* DC leaves showed higher polyphenol presence, antioxidant and antifungal activity and promoted cell proliferation in mice splenocytes." *An. Acad. Bras. Cienc.* 2019; 91(1): e20190916.

Bataglion, G., et al. "Determination of the phenolic composition from Brazilian tropical fruits by UHPLC-MS/MS." *Food Chem.* 2015 Aug; 180: 280–287.

Badejo, A., et al. "Gene expression of ascorbic acid biosynthesis related enzymes of the Smirnoff-Wheeler pathway in acerola (*Malpighia glabra*)." *J. Plant Physiol.* 2009 Apr; 166(6): 652–60.

Berni, P., et al. "Non-conventional tropical fruits: characterization, antioxidant potential and carotenoid bioaccessibility." *Plant Foods Hum. Nutr.* 2019 Mar; 74(1): 141–148.

Betta, F., et al "Phenolic compounds determined by LC-MS/MS and *in vitro* antioxidant capacity of Brazilian fruits in two edible ripening stages." *Plant Foods Hum. Nutr.* 2018 Dec; 73(4): 302–307.

Bowers, E., et al. "Vitamin C levels in old people and the response to ascorbic acid and to the juice of the acerola (*Malpighia punicifolia* L.). *Br. J. Clin. Pract.* 1965 Mar; 19: 141–147.

Cefali, L., et al. "Vitamin C in acerola and red plum extracts: Quantification via HPLC, *in vitro* antioxidant activity, and stability of their gel and emulsion. Formulations" *J. AOAC Int.* 2018 Sep; 101(5): 1461–1465.

Canuto, A., et al. "Physical and chemical characterization of fruit pulps from Amazonia and their correlation to free radical scavenger activity." 2010; 32(4): 1196–1205.

Chang, S., et al. "Superfruits: phytochemicals, antioxidant efficacies, and health effects – A comprehensive review." *Crit. Rev. Food Sci. Nutr.* 2018 Jan; 23: 1–25.

Correia, R., et al. "Bioactive compounds and phenolic-linked functionality of powdered tropical fruit residues." *Food Sci. Technol Int.* 2012 Dec; 18(6): 539–47.

Cruz, R., et al. "Comparison of the antioxidant property of acerola extracts with synthetic antioxidants using an *in vivo* method with yeasts." *Food Chem.* 2019 Mar; 277: 698–705.

Delva, L., et al. "Anthocyanin identification, vitamin C content, and antioxidant capacity of acerola (*Malpighia emarginata* DC) juices." *Proc. Fla. State Hort. Soc.* 2010; 123: 223–227.

Delva, L., "Acerola (*Malpighia emarginata* DC): Phenolic Profiling, Antioxidant Capacity, Antimicrobial Property, Toxicological Screening, and Color Stability." Dissertation. 2012 University of Florida, Food and Agricultural Sciences.

da Silva Nunes, R., et al. "Genotoxic and antigenotoxic activity of acerola (*Malpighia glabra* L.) extract in relation to the geographic origin." *Phytother. Res.* 2013 Oct; 27(10): 1495–501.

da Silva Nunes, et al. "Antigenotoxicity and antioxidant activity of acerola fruit (*Malpighia glabra* L.) at two stages of ripeness." *Food Chem.* 2011; 71:195–198.

de Brito, E., et al. "Anthocyanins present in selected tropical fruits: acerola, jambolao, jussara, and guajiru." *J. Agric. Food Chem.* 2007 Nov; 55(23): 9389–94.

de Assis, S., et al. "Antioxidant activity, ascorbic acid and total phenol of exotic fruits occurring in Brazil." *Int J. Food Sci. Nutr.* 2009 Aug; 60(5): 439–48.

de Rosso, V., et al. Determination of anthocyanins from acerola (*Malpighia emarginata* DC.) and açai (*Euterpe oleracea* Mart.) by HPLC–PDA–MS/MS." *J. Food Comp. Analy.* 2008 Jun; 21(4): 291–299.

Delva, L., et al. Antioxidant activity and antimicrobial properties of phenolic extracts from acerola (*Malpighia emarginata* DC) fruit." *Food Sci. Tech.* 2013 May; 48(5): 1048–1056.

Delva, L., et al. "Anthocyanin identification, vitamin C content, and antioxidant capacity of acerola (*Malpighia emarginata* DC) juices." *Proc. Fla. State Hort. Soc.* 2010; 123: 223–227.

Dusman, E., et al. "Radioprotective effect of the Barbados Cherry

(*Malpighia glabra* L.) against radiopharmaceutical iodine-131 in Wistar rats *in vivo.*" *BMC Complement. Altern. Med.* 2014 Jan; 14: 41.

Dusman, E., et al. "*In vivo* antimutagenic effects of the Barbados cherry fruit *(Malpighia glabra* Linnaeus) in a chromosomal aberration assay." *Genet. Mol. Res.* 2016 Dec; 15(4).

Hanamura, T., et al. "Structural and functional characterization of polyphenols isolated from acerola *(Malpighia emarginata* DC.) fruit." *Biosci. Biotechnol. Biochem.* 2005 Feb; 69(2): 280–6.

Hassimotto, N., et al. "Antioxidant activity of dietary fruits, vegetables, and commercial frozen fruit pulps." *J. Agric. Food Chem.* 2005 Apr 20; 53(8): 2928–35.

Horta, R. et al. "Protective effects of acerola juice on genotoxicity induced by iron *in vivo.*" *Genet. Mol. Biol.* 2016 Mar; 39(1): 122–8.

Klosterhoff, R., et al. "Structure and intracellular antioxidant activity of pectic polysaccharide from acerola *(Malpighia emarginata).*" *Int. J. Biol. Macromol.* 2018; 106: 473–480.

Leffa, D., et al. "Corrective effects of acerola *(Malpighia emarginata* DC.) juice intake on biochemical and genotoxical parameters in mice fed on a high-fat diet." *Mutat. Res.* 2014 Dec; 770: 144–52.

Lima, V., et al, "Antioxidant capacity of anthocyanins from acerola genotypes." *Food Sci. Tech.* 2011 Jan–Mar; 31(1): 86–92.

Marques, T., et al. "Phytochemicals from *Malpighia emarginata* rich in enzymatic inhibitor with modulatory action on hemostatic processes." *J. Food Sci.* 2018 Nov; 83(11): 2840–2849.

Marques, T. "Cereal bars enriched with antioxidant substances and rich in fiber, prepared with flours of acerola residues." *J. Food Sci. Technol.* 2015 Aug; 52(8): 5084–92.

Martinez, L., et al. "Green alternatives to synthetic antioxidants, antimicrobials, nitrates, and nitrites in clean label Spanish chorizo." *Antioxidants.* 2019 Jun 19; 8(6).

Mezadri, T., et al. "Antioxidant compounds and antioxidant activity in acerola *(Malpighia emarginata* DC.) fruits and derivatives." *J. Food Comp. Analy.* 2008; 21(4): 282–290.

Mezadri, T., et al. "Carotenoid pigments in acerola fruits *(Malpighia emarginata* DC.) and derived products." *EU Food Res. Tech.* 2005; 220: 63–69.

Motohashi, N., et al. "Biological activity of Barbados cherry (acerola fruits,

References

fruit of *Malpighia emarginata* DC) extracts and fractions." *Phytother. Res.* 2004 Mar; 18(3): 212–23.

Nascimento, E., et al "HPLC and *in vitro* evaluation of antioxidant properties of fruit from *Malpighia glabra* (Malpighiaceae) at different stages of maturation." *Food Chem. Toxicol.* 2018 Sep; 119: 457–463.

Neri-Numa, I., et al. "Small Brazilian wild fruits: Nutrients, bioactive compounds, health-promotion properties and commercial interest." *Food Res. Int.* 2018 Jan; 103: 345–360.

Nowak, D., et al. "Antioxidant properties and phenol compounds of vitamin C-rich juices." *J. Food Sci.* 2018 Aug; 83(8): 2237–2246.

Nunes, S., et al. "Antigenotoxicity and antioxidant activity of acerola fruit (*Malpighia glabra* L.) at two stages of ripeness." *Plant Foods Hum. Nutr.* 2011 Jun; 66(2) :129–35.

Oliveira, S., et al. "Antioxidant metabolism during fruit development of different acerola (*Malpighia emarginata* D.C) clones." *J. Agric. Food Chem.* 2012 Aug; 60(32): 7957–64.

Paz, M., et al. "Brazilian fruit pulps as functional foods and additives: evaluation of bioactive compounds." *Food Chem.* 2015 Apr 1; 172: 462–8.

Pereira, A., et al. "Synergistic, additive and antagonistic effects of fruit mixtures on total antioxidant capacities and bioactive compounds in tropical fruit juices." *Arch. Latinoam. Nutr.* 2015 Jun; 65(2): 119–27.

Prakash, A., et al. "Acerola, an untapped functional superfruit: A review on latest frontiers." *J. Food Sci. Technol.* 2018 Sep; 55(9): 3373–3384.

Ramalho, S., et al. "Evaluation of antioxidant capacity and L-ascorbic acid content in Brazilian tropical fruits acerola (*Malpighia emarginata*), mangaba (*Harconia speciosa*), siriguela (*Spondias purpurea*) and umbu (*Spondias tuberosa*)." *Planta Med.* 2011; 77: 200.

Righetto, A., et al. "Chemical composition and antioxidant activity of juices from mature and immature acerola (*Malpighia emarginata* DC)." 2005 Aug; 11(4): 315–321.

Rochette, N., et al. "Effect of the pretreatment with acerola (*Malpighia emarginata* DC.) juice on ethanol-induced oxidative stress in mice – Hepatoprotective potential of acerola juice." *Free Rad. Antioxid.* 2013 Dec; 3(Supl): S16–21.

Rufino, M., et al. "Bioactive compounds and antioxidant capacities of 18 non-traditional tropical fruits from Brazil." *Food Chemistry.* 2010 Aug; 121(4): 996–1002.

Rufino, M., et al. "Free radical-scavenging behaviour of some north-east Brazilian fruits in a DPPH system." *Food Chemistry* 2009 May; 114(2): 693–695.

Sagar, S., et al. "Estimation of physico-chemical properties, nutrient composition and antioxidant activity of acerola *Malpighia emarginata* DC." *J. Res. ANGRAU* 2013; 41(4): 97–101.

Sagar, S., et al. "Antioxidant properties of acerola (*Malpighia emarginata* DC.) and acerola squash." *Int. J. Sci. Res.* 2014 Jul; 3(7): 2176–2179.

Singh, D., et al. "Estimation of phytochemicals and antioxidant activity of underutilized fruits of Andaman Islands (India)." *Int. J. Food Sci. Nutr.* 2012; 63(4): 446–52.

Sousa, M., et al. "Antioxidant extract counteracts the effects of aging on cortical spreading depression and oxidative stress in the brain cortex." *Acta Cir. Bras.* 2018 Jun; 33(6): 472–482.

Sousa, K., et al. "Antioxidant compounds and total antioxidant activity in fruits of acerola from cv. Flor Branca, Florida Sweet and BRS 366." *Rev. Brasil. Fruitc.* 2014 Apr–Jun; 36(2): 294–304.

Visentainer, J., et al. "Physico-chemical characterization of acerola (*Malpighia glabra* L.) produced in Maringa, Parana State, Brazil." *Arch. Latinoam. Nutr.* 1997 Mar; 47(1): 70–2.

Visentainer, J., et al. "Vitamin C in Barbados cherry *Malpighia glabra* L. pulp submitted to processing and to different forms of storage." *Arch. Latinoam. Nutr.* 1998 Sep; 48(3): 256–9.

Wakabayashi, H., et al. "Inhibition of LPS-stimulated NO production in mouse macrophage-like cells by Barbados cherry, a fruit of *Malpighia emarginata* DC." *Anticancer Res.* 2003; 23(4): 3237–3241.

Xu, M., et al. "Metabolomic analysis of acerola cherry (*Malpighia emarginata*) fruit during ripening development via UPLC-Q-TOF and contribution to the antioxidant activity." *Food Res.* 2020 Apr; 130: 108915.

Chapter 7. More Benefits and Uses of Acerola

Heunks, l., et al. "Respiratory muscle function and free radicals: from cell to COPD." *Thorax.* 2000; 55: 704–716.

Reid, M. "Free radicals and muscle fatigue: Of ROS, canaries, and the IOC." *Free Radic. Biol. Med.* 2008 Jan; 44(2): 169–79.

Sousa, M., et al. "Antioxidant extract counteracts the effects of aging on cortical spreading depression and oxidative stress in the brain cortex." *Acta Cir. Bras.* 2018 Jun; 33(6): 472–482.

Thaler, J., et al. "Obesity is associated with hypothalamic injury in rodents and humans." *J. Clin. Invest.* 2012; 122: 153–162.

Anti-Aging and AGE-Inhibitor Actions

Hanamura, T., et al. "Structural and functional characterization of polyphenols isolated from acerola (*Malpighia emarginata* DC.) fruit." *Biosci. Biotech. Biochem.* 2004 Jul; 69: 280–286.

Yeh, W., et al. "Polyphenols with antiglycation activity and mechanisms of action: A review of recent findings." *J. Food. Drug. Anal.* 2017; 25: 84–92.

Anti-Allergy Actions

Ipci, K., et al. "Alternative products to treat allergic rhinitis and alternative routes for allergy immunotherapy." *Am. J. Rhinol. Allergy.* 2016 Sep; 30(5): 8–10.

Anticancer Actions

Dusman, E., et al. "*In vivo* antimutagenic effects of the Barbados cherry fruit (*Malpighia glabra* Linnaeus) in a chromosomal aberration assay." *Genet. Mol. Res.* 2016 Nov; 15(4): 15049036.

Motohashi, N., et al. "Biological activity of Barbados cherry (acerola fruits, fruit of *Malpighia emarginata* DC) extracts and fractions." *Phytother. Res.* 2004 Mar; 18(3): 212–23.

Nagamine, I., et al. "Effect of acerola cherry extract on cell proliferation and activation of RAS signal pathway at the promotion stage of lung tumorigenesis in mice." *J. Nutr. Sci. Vitaminol.* 2002 Feb; 48(1): 69–72.

Antidiabetic Actions

Barbalho, S., et al. "Evaluation of glycemic and lipid profile of offspring of diabetic Wistar rats treated with *Malpighia emarginata* juice." *Exp. Diabetes Res.* 2011; 2011: 173647.

Hanamura, T., et al. "Antihyperglycemic effect of polyphenols from Acerola (*Malpighia emarginata* DC.) fruit." *Biosci. Biotechnol. Biochem.* 2006 Aug; 70(8): 1813–20.

Hanamura, T., et al. "Structural and functional characterization of polyphenols isolated from acerola (*Malpighia emarginata* DC.) fruit." *Biosci. Biotech. Biochem.* 2004 Jul; 69: 280–286.

Kawaguichi, M., et al. "Isolation and characterization of a novel flavonoid possessing a 4,2''-glycosidic linkage from green mature acerola (*Malpighia emarginata* DC.) fruit." *Biosci. Biotechnol. Biochem.* 2007 May; 71(5): 1130–5.

Anti-Fatigue Actions

Klosterhoff, R., "Anti-fatigue activity of an arabinan-rich pectin from acerola *(Malpighia emarginata)*." *Int. J. Biol. Macromol.* 2018 Apr; 109: 1147–1153.

Azzolino, D., et al. "Nutritional status as a mediator of fatigue and its underlying mechanisms in older people." *Nutrients.* 2020 Feb; 12(2): E444.

Pastor, R., et al. "Response to exercise in older adults who take supplements of antioxidants and/or omega-3 polyunsaturated fatty acids: A systematic review." *Biochem. Pharmacol.* 2019 Oct 3: 113649. [ahead of print]

Antimicrobial Actions

Barros, B., et al. "Saline extract from *Malpighia emarginata* DC leaves showed higher polyphenol presence, antioxidant and antifungal activity and promoted cell proliferation in mice splenocytes." *An. Acad. Bras. Cienc.* 2019; 91(1): e20190916.

Caceres, A., et al. "Plants used in Guatemala for the treatment of dermatophytic infections. 2. Evaluation of antifungal activity of seven American plants." *J. Ethnopharmacol.* 1993 Dec; 40(3): 207–13.

Delva, L., et al. Antioxidant activity and antimicrobial properties of phenolic extracts from acerola (*Malpighia emarginata* DC) fruit." *Food Sci. Tech.* 2013 May; 48(5): 1048–1056.

Martinez, L., et al. "Green alternatives to synthetic antioxidants, antimicrobials, nitrates, and nitrites in clean label Spanish chorizo." *Antioxidants.* 2019 Jun 19; 8(6).

Motohashi, N., et al. "Biological activity of Barbados cherry (acerola fruits, fruit of *Malpighia emarginata* DC) extracts and fractions." *Phytother. Res.* 2004 Mar; 18(3): 212–23.

Oliveira, A., et al. "Microbial control and quorum sensing inhibition by phenolic compounds of acerola (*Malpighia emarginata*)." *Intl. Food. Res. J.* 2017 Oct; 4(5): 2228–2237.

Silva L., et al. "Delivery of phytochemicals of tropical fruit by-products using poly (DL-lactide-co-glycolide) (PLGA) nanoparticles: synthesis, characterization, and antimicrobial activity." *Food Chem.* 2014 Dec; 165: 362–70.

References

Tremonte, P., et al. "Antimicrobial effect of *Malpighia punicifolia* and extension of water buffalo steak shelf-life." *J. Food Sci.* 2016 Jan; 81(1): M97-105.

Anti-Obesity Actions

Dias, F., et al. "Acerola (*Malpighia emarginata* DC.) juice intake protects against alterations to proteins involved in inflammatory and lipolysis pathways in the adipose tissue of obese mice fed a cafeteria diet." *Lipids Health Dis.* 2014 Feb 4; 13: 24.

Hanamura, T., et al. "Structural and functional characterization of polyphenols isolated from acerola (*Malpighia emarginata* DC.) fruit." *Biosci. Biotech. Biochem.* 2004 Jul; 69: 280–286.

Hu, Y., et al. "Acerola polysaccharides ameliorate high-fat diet-induced non-alcoholic fatty liver disease through reduction of lipogenesis and improvement of mitochondrial functions in mice." *Food Funct.* 2020; 11: 1037–1048.

Kawaguichi, M., et al. "Isolation and characterization of a novel flavonoid possessing a 4,2''-glycosidic linkage from green mature acerola (*Malpighia emarginata* DC.) fruit." *Biosci. Biotechnol. Biochem.* 2007 May; 71(5): 1130–5.

Leffa, D., et al. "Corrective effects of acerola (*Malpighia emarginata* DC.) juice intake on biochemical and genotoxical parameters in mice fed on a high-fat diet." *Mutat. Res.* 2014 Dec; 770: 144–52.

Leffa, D., et al. "Effects of acerola (*Malpighia emarginata* DC.) juice intake on brain energy metabolism of mice fed a cafeteria diet." *Mol. Neurobiol.* 2017 Mar; 54(2): 954–963.

Leffa, D., et al. "Effects of supplemental acerola juice on the mineral concentrations in liver and kidney tissue samples of mice fed with cafeteria diet." *Biol. Trace Elem. Res.* 2015 Sep; 167(1): 70–6.

Marques, T., et al. "Methanolic extract of *Malpighia emarginata* bagasse: phenolic compounds and inhibitory potential on digestive enzymes." *Rev. Bras. Farmacogn.* 2016 Mar/Apr: 25(2): 191–196.

Mezadri, T., et al. "The acerola fruit: composition, productive characteristics and economic importance." *Arch. Latinoam. Nutr.* 2006 Jun; 56(2): 101–9.

Cholesterol-Lowering Actions

Barbalho, S., et al. "Evaluation of glycemic and lipid profile of offspring of diabetic Wistar rats treated with *Malpighia emarginata* juice." *Exp. Diabetes Res.* 2011; 2011: 173647.

Batista, K., et al. "Beneficial effects of consumption of acerola, cashew or guava processing by-products on intestinal health and lipid metabolism in dyslipidaemic female Wistar rats." *Br. J. Nutr.* 2018 Jan; 119(1): 30–41.

Benefits For the Skin

Gause, S., et al. "UV-blocking potential of oils and juices." *Int. J. Cosmet. Sci.* 2016 Aug; 38(4): 354–63.

Hanamura, T., et al. "Skin-lightening effect of a polyphenol extract from acerola (*Malpighia emarginata* DC.) fruit on UV-induced pigmentation." *Biosci. Biotechnol. Biochem.* 2008 Dec; 72(12): 3211–8.

Kawaguchi, M. "*Acerola Fruit-Derived Pectin and Its Application.*" US Patent No. 20080267894. October 30, 2008.

Sato, Y., et al. "Juice intake suppresses UVB-induced skin pigmentation in SMP30/GNL knockout hairless mice." *PLoS One.* 2017 Jan; 12(1): e0170438.

Chapter 8. A Consumer Guide for Acerola

Safety/Nontoxic Actions

Belwal, T., et al. "Phytopharmacology of acerola (*Malpighia spp.*) and its potential as functional food." *Trends Food Sci. Tech.* 2018 Apr; 74: 99–106.

Chang, S., et al. "Superfruits: phytochemicals, antioxidant efficacies, and health effects - A comprehensive review." *Crit. Rev. Food Sci. Nutr.* 2018 Jan; 23: 1–25.

da Silva Nunes, R., et al. "Genotoxic and antigenotoxic activity of acerola (*Malpighia glabra* L.) extract in relation to the geographic origin." *Phytother. Res.* 2013 Oct; 27(10): 1495–501.

Delva, L., "Acerola (*Malpighia emarginata* DC): phenolic profiling, antioxidant capacity, antimicrobial property, toxicological screening, and color stability." Dissertation. 2012 University of Florida, Food and Agricultural Sciences.

Hanamura, T., et al. "Toxicological evaluation of polyphenol extract from acerola (*Malpighia emarginata* DC.) fruit." *J. Food Sci.* 2008 May; 73(4): T55–61.

Johnson, P. "Acerola (*Malpighia glabra* L., *M. punicifolia* L., *M. emarginata* D.C.): agriculture, production and nutrition." *World Rev. Nutr. Diet.* 2003; 91: 67–75.

Prakash, A., and Baskaran, R. "Acerola, an untapped functional superfruit: a review on latest frontiers." *J. Food Sci. Technol.* 2018 Sep; 55(9): 3373–3384.

References

Processing and Manufacturing Methods

Alves Filho, E., et al. "Evaluation of thermal and non-thermal processing effect on non-prebiotic and prebiotic acerola juices using (1)H qNMR and GC-MS coupled to chemometrics." *Food Chem.* 2018 Nov; 265: 23–31.

Benjamin, S., et al. "Electroanalysis for quality control of acerola (*Malpighia emarginata*) fruits and their commercial products." *Food Anal. Methods* 2015; 8: 86–92.

Caetano, A., et al. "Evaluation of antioxidant activity of agro-industrial waste of acerola (*Malpighia emarginata* DC) fruit extracts." *Food Sci. Tech.* 2011 Jul–Sep; 31(3): 769–775.

De Moraes, F., et al. "Freeze dried acerola (*Malpighia emarginata*) pulp and pomace: physicochemical attributes, phytochemical content and stability during storage." *J. Food Indust.* 2017; Vol. 1(1): 17–38.

Delva, L., et al. "Acerola (*Malpighia emarginata* DC): production, postharvest handling, nutrition, and biological activity." *Food Rev. Intern.* 2013; 29(2): 107–126.

Duzzioni, A., et al. "Effect of drying kinetics on main bioactive compounds and antioxidant activity of acerola (*Malpighia emarginata* DC) residue." Food Sci. Tech. 2013 May; 48(5): 1041–1047.

Eca, K., et al. "Development of active films from pectin and fruit extracts: light protection, antioxidant capacity, and compounds stability." *J. Food Sci.* 2015 Nov; 80(11): C2389–96.

Krishnaiah, D., et al. "A critical review on the spray drying of fruit extract: effect of additives on physicochemical properties." *Crit. Rev. Food Sci. Nutr.* 2014; 54(4): 449–73.

Kuivanen, J., et al. "Metabolic engineering of the fungal D-galacturonate pathway for L-ascorbic acid production." *Microb. Cell. Fact.* 2015 Jan; 14: 2.

Marques, T., et al. "Chemical constituents and technological functional properties of acerola (*Malpighia emarginata* DC.) waste flour." *Food Sci. Technol.* 2013 Oct; 33(3): 526–531.

Marques, T., et al. "Fruit bagasse phytochemicals from *Malpighia emarginata* rich in enzymatic inhibitor with modulatory action on hemostatic processes." *J. Food Sci.* 2018 Nov; 83(11): 2840–2849.

Marques, L., et al. "Freeze-drying of acerola (*Malpighia glabra* L.)." *Chem. Eng. Process. Process Intense.* 2007 May; 46(5): 451–457.

Mercali, G., et al. "Degradation kinetics of anthocyanins in acerola pulp:

comparison between ohmic and conventional heat treatment." *Food Chem.* 2013 Jan; 136(2): 853–7.

Mercali, G., et al. "Study of vitamin C degradation in acerola pulp during ohmic and conventional heat treatment." *Food. Sci. Tech.* 2012 Jun; 47(1): 91–95.

Oliveira, L., et al. "The influence of processing and long-term storage on the antioxidant metabolism of acerola (*Malpighia emarginata*) purée." *Braz. J. Plant Physiol.,* 2011; 23(2): 151–160.

Ribeiro da Silva, L., et al. "Quantification of bioactive compounds in pulps and by-products of tropical fruits from Brazil." *Food Chem.* 2014 Jan; 143: 398–404.

Ribeiro, H., et al. "Stabilizing effect of montmorillonite on acerola juice anthocyanins." *Food Chem.* 2018 Apr; 245: 966–973.

Santos, V., et al. "Improvements on the stability and vitamin content of acerola juice obtained by ultrasonic processing." *Foods.* 2018 May; 7(5): E68.

Silva, P., et al. "A novel system for drying of agro-industrial acerola (*Malpighia emarginata* DC) waste for use as bioactive compound source." *Innov. Food Sci. Emerg. Technol.* 2019 Mar; 52: 350–357.

Silva, P., et al. "Dehydration of acerola (*Malpighia emarginata* DC) residue in a new designed rotary dryer: Effect of process variables on main bioactive compounds." *Food Bioprod. Process.* 2016 Apr; 98: 62–70.

Souza, C., et al. "Mango and acerola pulps as antioxidant additives in cassava starch bio-based film." *J. Agric. Food Chem.* 2011 Mar; 59(6): 2248–54.

Wurlitzer, N., et al. "Tropical fruit juice: effect of thermal treatment and storage time on sensory and functional properties." *J. Food Sci. Technol.* 2019 Dec; 56(12): 5184–5193.

About the Author

Leslie Taylor is one of the world's leading experts on rainforest medicinal plants. She founded, managed, and directed the Raintree group of companies from 1995 to 2012, and was a leader in creating a worldwide market for the important medicinal plants of the Amazon rainforest.

Having survived a rare form of leukemia only because of alternative health and herbal medicine, Leslie has been researching, studying, and documenting alternative healing modalities—including herbal medicine—for more than thirty years. A dedicated herbalist and naturopath, she developed many herbal formulas and remedies for her companies, for practitioners, and for individuals needing help. In 1995, while researching alternative AIDS and cancer therapies in Europe, Leslie became aware of a medicinal plant from the Peruvian rainforest called cat's claw. This research took her to the Peruvian rainforest to gain firsthand knowledge about this new medicinal plant. Upon her return, she founded Raintree Nutrition, Inc., to make this important rainforest medicinal plant and others available in the United States.

After that first trip, Leslie returned to the Amazon numerous times, continuing to research and document more rainforest medicinal plants. In these endeavors, she worked directly with indigenous Indian shamans and healers, learning about their use of healing plants, as well as with indigenous tribal communities and other rainforest communities. She also worked with phytochemists, botanists, ethnobotanists, researchers, and alternative and integrative health practitioners to document, research, test, and validate rainforest medicinal plants.

In 2012, with many other companies selling the rainforest plants that she had introduced to the United States, she decided to close her business and naturopathic practice and devote herself to educating people about the benefits of medicinal plants. She freely shared all her proprietary formulas by posting them on the Raintree website so that anyone can make and use them.

Now, Leslie Taylor remains a trusted source of factual information about rainforest medicinal plants and continues to update the Tropical Plant Database for these purposes. A practicing board certified naturopath for many years (now retired), she has lectured and taught classes in naturopathic medicine, herbal medicine, and ethnobotany, as well as environmental and sustainability issues in the Amazon rainforest. She is the author of *Herbal Secrets of the Rainforest* and of the best-selling *The Healing Power of Rainforest Herbs*, as well as the highly popular and extensively referenced Raintree Tropical Plant Database (http://www.rain-tree.com/plants.htm), which has been online since 1996.

More information about Leslie Taylor and her other books can be found at http://rain-tree.com/author.htm and on her Amazon Author Page. She also has a personal blog where you can ask questions and share your results using acerola with others at http://leslie-taylor-raintree.blogspot.com/acerola.html.